# MENOPAUSE AND BEYOND

## HOW TO CONTROL EMOTIONS, BEAT HOT FLASHES, ACHIEVE RESTFUL SLEEP, LOSE BELLY WEIGHT, AND AGE GRACEFULLY WITH CONFIDENCE

### KATE HARTWELL

# CONTENTS

# INTRODUCTION

What's the first thing that comes to mind when you hear the word *menopause*? Trust me, whatever comes to your mind is valid, as we all have certain ideas about what we think or imagine menopause to be. Most of what we think about menopause probably comes from what we see in the media or what we have heard from other women around us, those who may have already gone through it, or those who are right in the thick of it.

I hope that this book is going to answer all the questions you have on this subject. Before we even begin, I want to declare this a judgment-free zone, where you can come up with all your preconceived ideas and opinions about menopause and weigh them against what you learn here. The menopause journey is personal and unique to each woman, so no two women will go through exactly the same experience of it. The aim of this book is to provide some guidance for women who are going through this beautiful phase of life by providing both factual information and practical strategies to help them navigate certain aspects of it.

As you approach menopause, you may have questions and concerns. One of these could be a deep-seated fear of losing your identity, especially when you start experiencing both physical and psychological symptoms, some of which could leave you in a position where you do not recognize yourself anymore. Have you started experiencing hot flashes, night sweats, and sleep disturbances? If so, these could be unpredictable and intense. When this happens, it could cause discomfort and disrupt your daily routines. Also, as your hormones start fluctuating, this could bring about mood swings, anxiety, and depression. These emotional shifts can be confusing and distressing, making you feel unlike your usual self. Maybe you have noticed that you are slowly losing interest in sex. This is something that would strain the relationship with your partner, and when this happens, it could affect your self-esteem.

Your body may also start going through visible physical changes; maybe you have started gaining some weight and are noticing some loss of skin elasticity. To make matters worse, as women, we suffer a lot from societal pressures around youth, being expected to maintain our looks forever, and these changes could make you feel insecure about your body and age. This usually leads to a decrease in self-confidence and heightened self-consciousness.

If you are going through some or all of the above, you are not alone, so go easy on yourself. You are already doing something about it, and I believe you are here because you've got questions and are wondering if this book can provide the answers and guidance that you are looking for.

Well, the answer is simple. In this book, you will learn the Radiant Shift Method—a method that invites you, the reader, to explore menopause in a new light. It will help you reframe your experiences and encourage you to see menopause not as an ending or a decline but as a vibrant transition into a new phase of life with its own strengths and potential. While many solutions focus primarily on alleviating the physical symptoms of menopause, Radiant Shift goes beyond symptom management. It challenges the prevalent negative narratives about menopause, reframes them, and positions menopause not as an ending but as a powerful phase of growth and transformation.

The book presents all of this information in carefully structured and easy-to-understand chapters that cover the following areas:

*Chapter 1:*

Redefining menopause - In this chapter, we discuss the cultural and historical narratives surrounding menopause.

*Chapter 2:*

The Full Spectrum - Here, we explore the variety and depth of menopausal symptoms to help you understand the holistic experience of menopause.

*Chapter 3:*

Tides of Emotion - In this chapter, we discuss the emotional changes that accompany menopause and will empower you with the techniques for harnessing those emotional shifts.

*Chapter 4:*

A New Dawn of Intimacy - Here, we explore the nuances of sexuality during menopause. This chapter aims to show you how to embrace and redefine your sensuality and discover renewed confidence and self-appreciation.

*Chapter 5:*

Bridging Wisdom -In this chapter, we delve into the intersection between modern medical approaches and traditional remedies for managing menopause. You will learn about various treatments and discover the potential benefits of a holistic approach.

*Chapter 6:*

A Radiant Life - In this chapter, we talk about the crucial role of lifestyle during menopause. Here, you will learn to incorporate holistic practices into your life, fostering greater balance and joy during menopause.

*Chapter 7:*

A Journey Inward - This chapter explores the philosophical aspect of menopause. Here, you will learn how to embrace life during and after menopause.

*Chapter 8:*

Being a Pillar - This chapter is a bonus chapter for those who play the crucial role of a supporter in a woman's menopausal journey. Supporters will learn practical and empathetic approaches to aid menopausal women in their lives here.

With that said, I can't wait to dive in and put it all into context in Chapter 1.

# 1

# REDEFINING MENOPAUSE

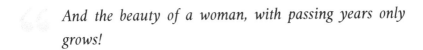

*And the beauty of a woman, with passing years only grows!*

— AUDREY HEPBURN

## THE HISTORY OF MENOPAUSE

The word *menopause* has its roots in ancient Greece—*men* in Greek means the month and the moon, and *pauein* means to stop or cease, thus meaning the end of the monthly cycle for the woman. The term itself was created by a French physician, Dr. Charles Negrier, in 1821 (Moore, 2020). Since life spans were much shorter back in the olden days, with very few women living past the age of 40, there isn't much literature on menopause as a subject of inquiry in those times. Over time, interest in this stage of life began to pique; however, menopause was regarded as a natural part of life. Sometime in the early nineteenth century, there was a shift toward viewing menopause as a medical phenomenon, as doctors started searching for ways to treat the symptoms accompanying this condition using science.

## THE CULTURAL NARRATIVE

As we look at the history of menopause, it is important that we also look at it from a cultural perspective. What we know is that the West views menopause very differently from how other cultures view it. Take the Japanese; for instance, the word *konenki* in Japanese is the word for menopause, and what it breaks down to is *ko* for "renewal and regeneration," *nen* for "years," and *ki* for "season or energy" (Women's Health Network, 2023). You can clearly see how positively they view this phase of a woman's life—a season to be embraced rather than dreaded. Even the Chinese call it the "Second Spring." Spring has a positive connotation; it's a season of renewal. It wasn't even until recently that the Japanese coined a term for hot flashes, as previously they did not have this in their vocabulary. This is simply because this was not a thing for most women in their culture. It is estimated that only about 25% of Japanese women experience hot flashes (Women's Health Network, 2023). The words *hotto furasshur* for "hot flash" and *horumon baransu* for "hormone balance" were created for the Japanese to communicate with Western media on this subject (Women's Health Network, 2023). Even the way Japanese women manage the process when they experience the symptoms of menopause is very different, as most don't opt for hormone replacement.

Diet could play a significant role in the variation of symptoms across different cultures with a diet low in fiber and high in bad fats, as is common in North America, suspected to contribute hugely to hormonal imbalances.

Another fascinating culture that experiences menopause differently and with a positive outlook that is similar to the Japanese is the Mayans. Mayan women report fewer experiences with the dreaded menopause symptoms that are common among Western women. Though they show similar follicle-stimulating hormone (FSH) blood levels as North American women, they seem to have very low incidences of osteoporosis, similar to Japanese women. In short, FSHs are the follicles that control women's menstrual cycle and the growth of eggs. Mayan women also report looking forward to menopause, as for them, reaching this stage of life is tied to acquiring a new status in the community where they can become spiritual leaders. So this is a stage that is often embraced in this culture. Other possible explanations for these cultural differences include geography, diet, lifestyle, and genetics, of course.

When we trace the history of menopause, we see how menopause has become medicalized over the years, especially in the West, where instead of treating it as a natural stage of life, it is now treated as a disease. This is a stark difference from how the other cultures that we have discussed above approach it. This was not always the case, though, as Waltz (2021) points out that it was the Age of Enlightenment in Ancient Europe that brought about the shift to viewing menopause and women's sexual health negatively.

According to Waltz (2021), the medical community incorrectly believed that women's minds were controlled by their ovaries, something they believed made women susceptible to insanity. This resulted in menopause being demonized, along with the symptoms that accompanied it. Women who experienced depression, anxiety, restlessness, and sleeplessness were diagnosed with a condition called "climacteric insanity" or hysteria. The result of that? Some women were being locked up in asylums and, in worst-case scenarios, having their ovaries removed if they were deemed "diseased," all in an effort to cure them of this condition. Did you know that even the word "hysteria" comes from the Greek word *hystera*, a word for uterus?

More recently, in the 1930s, medical research on menopause started gaining traction as the medical community began viewing it as a disease of hormone deficiency, and in the 1970s, they started prescribing hormone replacement therapy (HRT). This happened after Thelma and Robert Wilson, a gynecologist and his wife, wrote a book called *Feminine Forever*, a book that called menopause a disease of estrogen deficiency, which, according to the pair, robbed women of their femininity and quality of life (Moore, 2020).

Dr. Robert A. Wilson wrote (Murtagh & Hepworth, 2003):

> *The unpalatable truth must be faced that all post-menopausal women are castrates... Our streets abound with them – walking stiffly in twos and threes, seeing little and observing less. It is not unusual to see an erect man of 75 vigorously striding along on a golf course, but never a woman of this age... Now, for the first time in history, women may share the*

*promise of tomorrow as biological equals of men. Thanks to hormone therapy, they can be feminine forever. (p. 187)*

Today, some scientists are against the medication for menopause. One such group is led by Dr. Martha Hickey from the Royal Women's Hospital in Australia, who argues that medicalizing menopause risks reducing a wide range of experiences from different women into a defined disease that requires treatment and that it often overemphasizes the negative aspects of it (Munsi, n.d.). In her book, *The Estrogen Elixir: A History of Hormone Replacement in America*, Elizabeth Siegel Watkins (2007) argues that the manner in which scientists are approaching the treatment of menopause is a reflection of today's culture in regards to middle-aged women. In this book, she specifically mentions UCLA professor Dr. Shelton, who touted long-term HRT as something that would help women maintain their youthful appearance, happy marriages, and positive attitude, over and above the benefit of preventing osteoporosis.

The media has also done its fair share in promoting HRT, a trend that started in the '40s with popular magazines like *Ladies' Home Journal* or *Good Housekeeping*, which initially tried to encourage women to accept this stage of life as something "not to be feared but embraced." When more popular magazines like *Vogue*, *Harper's Bazaar*, and *Newsweek* jumped on this bandwagon of discussing menopause as a subject, menopause became more and more seen as a disease to be medicated rather than a natural stage of life. It was during these times that pharmaceutical companies started using the media to advertise and sell HRT, especially because, in those days, women often looked at magazines as sources of information and advice.

Before that, pharmaceutical companies had been promoting heavily in the doctors' rooms with pamphlets and posters and getting medics to write opinion pieces.

HRT was promoted as a pill that plays a vital role in preventing aging, which can help women live longer and happier lives, and with the promotion of HRT, menopause was seen as something to be avoided or dreaded. Even though there were a few people who were cautioning against the quick adoption of a pill as a "cure-all" and issuing a warning that there is no pill that can reset the clock, HRT continued to gain popularity amongst hordes of women who just wanted the symptoms to go away. Gorrepati (2019) talks about how it wasn't until 1975 that HRT started receiving negative press when data from two medical studies showed a possible link to endometrial cancers. Not only was this information discussed in medical circles, but popular media sources like the *New York Times* got wind of it and ran the story. According to Gorrepati (2019), the case against HRT was strengthened even more when a study done by the Women's Health Initiative was stopped prematurely by the US government in 2002 due to preliminary data that showed an increase in blood clots, breast cancer, stroke, and heart disease. The aim of that study was to investigate the risks and benefits of HRT in preventing diseases. This came as a definite shock to many, who were left wondering why things had been allowed to go that far in viewing menopause as a disease to the point of medicalizing it.

## HOW HAVE SOCIETAL EXPERIENCES SHAPED WOMEN'S EXPERIENCES?

### How the Media Portrays Menopause

When it comes to print media, a study that reviewed close to 3,000 articles published in the UK over the last decade showed that there was increased interest in the media about this phase of life. Sadly, however, the results also showed that an overwhelming majority of articles tended to portray menopause in a negative light (Rowson et al., 2023). The researchers reported that menopause was often shown as a stage of dysfunction, unpredictable behavior from a woman, and decline, which further perpetuated the stigma that women in menopause are the "dangerous other, affected by both physical and mental abnormalities."

More than a quarter (27%) of UK women 50 years old and above feel that advertisements in the media contribute to creating and maintaining a negative stereotype of their age group (Marketing Communication News, 2018). In fact, the majority of women in this study felt that ads failed to address the issue of menopause with any sensitivity, often presenting women of this age as frumpy or clueless when it comes to technology. This study also revealed that menopausal women feel that society expects them to just vanish from public life as they age. A quarter of these women reported that this caused them to lose their confidence and that it had negatively impacted their relationships.

It's not like TV shows are doing a better job. Shows from the '70s up until now haven't done much to give a better perspective on menopausal women. In fact, according to McCullough (2019), how the media, specifically TV shows, portrays menopause is not only misleading but potentially harmful. She asserts that most of them promote the fallacy that menopause operates like a switch, taking a woman by surprise when she wakes up one day and discovers that she's at that stage. These shows never mention perimenopause, which could last for years, or its accompanying symptoms. A beautiful illustration of this point is found in one episode of *The Golden Girls,* where one of the characters thinks she's pregnant but learns that, in fact, she's in menopause. In another show called *All in the Family,* one of the main characters is portrayed as volatile and erratic in behavior, and that's when she discovers that she's going through "the change" and her "poor" husband has to put up with the changes. More recently, in the Netflix show Dead to Me, the character that plays Judy Hale is disappointed to learn that she's not pregnant but is in menopause, again pushing the narrative that all women have this desire to reproduce and that they often tie their worth to their ability to do so. Instead of viewing menopause as a relief from heavy menses, this highlights the negative side of losing the ability to reproduce.

All in all, what we are seeing is that both print and digital media are perpetuating the "aging woman" stereotype that menopausal women are irritable, unattractive, and mentally and emotionally unstable. Most show women as insecure, frazzled, and desperately trying to cling to their youth (Anderson, 2021).

When it comes to the workplace, there isn't much support there either, but rather a misconception that menopausal women are less productive or capable in the workplace. This has been proven to be false. A recent study showed that women leaders excelled during the COVID-19 crisis, confirming what previous research had shown about women leaders (Stillman, 2021). This article uses the example of New Zealand Prime Minister Jacinda Ardern, who managed to keep her country almost COVID-free during the pandemic. These researchers also combed through a database of more than 60,000 reviews of business leaders assessing how business executives fared during the crisis, and women came out on top, showing that women leaders perform better during a crisis.

It has been estimated that ageism could cost the US $63 billion in health costs alone (Gaskell, 2023). Sadly, aging doesn't affect men and women equally but is rather more unfair to women. A study from Berkeley-Haas showed that male professors were assessed more favorably than female professors, whose scores peaked when they were in their 30s and fell harshly in their mid-to-late 40s. Female professors were seen as less warm, a definite gendered societal norm for females. What is troubling is that women are expected to constantly adapt to changing societal expectations, which is something that affects women psychologically as they often suffer from burnout while trying to constantly rise to expectations. Prof. Chatman, who experienced this firsthand at the university, mentioned how deeply entrenched gender stereotypes are. She mentioned that even when similar information was provided about a male and a female professor, the female would still score lower than a male counterpart. This led to the conclusion that females are expected to subscribe to the stereotypical notions of being "nice" and "warm" even while climbing the proverbial ladder career-wise.

## MENOPAUSE THROUGH THE FEMINIST LENS

There is a raging debate that's currently going on about whether to go for hormone therapy or to treat menopause as a natural phenomenon that doesn't need to be medicalized. There is a strong feminist voice that has taken a stand against medicalizing menopause. Basically, there are two camps. On the one hand, we have feminists advocating that menopause is a natural phase of life to be perceived as bringing us freedom from the shackles of being viewed as sex objects. And what about the great relief from menses, right? Feminists are rejecting the patriarchal notion of determining a woman's worth based on their ability to reproduce. This makes it look like the end of a woman's reproductive cycle pronounces a death sentence for the woman—the end of their productive life. This is a group that advocates for the use of natural supplements, vitamins, herbs, yoga, and acupuncture. On the other hand, we have pharmaceutical companies and doctors asking why you go through all that suffering when you can get relief from HRT. These guys are promising not only relief from the symptoms, but they are also peddling HRT as a fountain of youth, which is a great selling point, I would say.

This debate is almost similar to the one about natural birth versus using drugs. It seems there is always going to be a division between those who approach certain stages of life as natural phenomena that should be embraced, warts and all, and those who say, why suffer when you can medicalize? I personally don't believe one group is superior to the other, as we all go through these experiences as individuals with different needs, and making a selfish decision when you're faced with one isn't a bad thing. It seems women are always going to be haunted by what Warrick (1994) describes as a "fear of selling out the sisterhood," but ultimately, you have to do what is right for you. In her article, she gives examples of women who swore not to sell out but, changed their minds when things got rough.

Most feminists want women to view and embrace menopause as an art and an opportunity to enjoy the freedom that comes with being non-sexual. There is a lot of truth in that as this view, in my opinion, empowers women to make it a positive experience instead of something that should be feared and "treated."

## RE-IMAGINING MENOPAUSE: IT IS NOT THE END

At this point, I want to invite you to join me as we collectively shift our perspective as women to view menopause not as an end to something, as is widely purported in the media, but as the beginning of a beautiful phase of life that should be embraced positively. Menopause is not a problem that needs to be solved. In her article, *The Midlife Unraveling*, where she shares her experiences of approaching midlife, Dr. Brene Brown (2018) talks about the point at which she realized that attaching the label "crisis" to it was, in her own words, "bullshit".

This demonstrates the power of a positive mindset—that when we shift from expecting the negative to focusing on the positive, we will have a very different experience. She proposes that maybe it's time we let go of all the fear and shame we've been carrying from our younger years and embrace love at this stage.

I love Jen Gunter's suggestion too, where she says, "Think of menopause as crossing the crimson bridge, a planned biological change that has been a vital contributor to the evolution of humankind" (Gunter, 2021). She reminds us that menopause has always been labeled as frailty or weakness, simply because that was the narrative of the patriarchy of the ancient days. Instead, she urges us, women, to own the story of agency and voice, value, and find the knowledge that will keep us in the healthiest condition as we continue to ask for what is rightfully ours, the proverbial "seat at the table."

A large part of why menopause is viewed with fear is because most women don't know what to expect from it; in some cultures, it's still a taboo subject, and even those who are already going through it don't really talk about their experiences. This could be addressed by holding educational programs and awareness workshops around the world, not just for women but for their families too. Many of the false narratives could be addressed during these sessions, and women could be educated about the beauty of this phase of life and given the tools to take care of themselves as they go through "the change."

CONCLUSION

In this chapter, we traced the history of menopause and spoke about how different cultures approach it. Throughout the chapter, the message is crisp and clear: menopause is what you make it, and it's a very personal and unique experience for each woman who goes through it. In concluding this chapter, I want to reiterate what I have been saying for the most part—that menopause is not to be feared or approached with angst, anxiety, or the shame of losing your youth. Just by shifting your attitude to a more positive one and grabbing this opportunity with both hands as an opportunity for a do-over, you can have a totally different experience. By that, what I mean is: use it to do everything you wish you could have done in your younger years—travel, take care of your body, learn a new skill, or take up a hobby. If you do this, you will definitely have a rewarding experience that offers personal fulfillment and growth. This is the "Radiant Shift."

But perhaps the best place to start is by arming ourselves with knowledge, to learn as much as we can about menopause, what it is, the symptoms, and all the ins and outs, and this next chapter will cover all of that.

# 2

# THE FULL SPECTRUM

66 *You have to sit down and take a good look at yourself, particularly as you grow older and your face changes. People are afraid of changing; that they're losing something. They don't understand that they are also gaining something.*

— SHARON STONE

## WHAT IS MENOPAUSE?

Menopause officially happens once a woman has gone for 12 consecutive months without menstruating. This is triggered by a shift in hormones that takes place as the body approaches the end of its reproductive years. On average, menopause happens around age 52 in the US (Office on Women's Health, 2019). Most women report experiencing hot flashes, night sweats, and weight changes as the most common symptoms of menopause, so these are the most well-known symptoms, but there are others that we will talk about a bit later. Menopause is a process that happens in stages and can often start approximately four years before the last period occurs, with symptoms happening over several years. Even though the process may be the same, the experience will certainly be different from one woman to the next and unique to each one.

## PERIMENOPAUSE

Perimenopause means "around" menopause, and it simply means the time that leads up to your last period (Office on Women's Health, 2019). Many women start experiencing the symptoms during this time, and that's why it is regarded as the "transition period." The transition period can be any length of time, even up to ten years for some women, and usually, it begins when a woman is in her 40s. What happens during this time is that the ovaries start producing less estrogen, and when this drop in estrogen accelerates, you may begin to experience the symptoms of menopause, usually in the last year or two before the actual onset of menopause. It's very important to remember that you can still get pregnant during this time.

You may hear people talking about early menopause, which is when a woman goes into menopause in her 40s, usually between 45 and 50 years old. Research shows that about five percent of women experience this (Office on Women's Health, 2019). Lifestyle factors such as smoking and certain medications can trigger the early onset of menopause. Some women also experience what is called premature menopause or primary ovarian insufficiency, a condition when menopause happens before one turns 40 years old.

## MENOPAUSE

As already mentioned earlier, this is the official end of your reproductive years, a stage that a woman reaches after 12 consecutive months of not menstruating. You reach this stage when your ovaries stop releasing eggs and producing most of their estrogen (Cleveland Clinic, 2021).

## POSTMENOPAUSE

Once you have gone for an entire year since the official start of your menopause and all through the rest of your life, you can now say that you are postmenopausal. Even though the menopause symptoms will get better postmenopause, some women report that they still experience hot flashes and other menopause symptoms for up to a decade, or even longer. Your risk of conditions like osteoporosis may increase at this stage due to lowered estrogen production.

## WHY DOES MENOPAUSE HAPPEN?

Normal menopause happens as part of the aging process. By normal, I'm talking about menopause that is not caused by surgery or any type of medical intervention, such as the removal of one's ovaries. This process takes place over time, as I mentioned under the perimenopause stage. Around this time, some of the changes that start happening in your body pertain to how it produces hormones like estrogen and progesterone, as well as other hormones. The said changes happen because your body loses active ovarian follicles, the structures responsible for producing and releasing eggs (Huizen, 2023). During this time, your ovaries will also start slowing down the production of estrogen, which directly affects the menstrual cycle. Your cycle may become irregular and will eventually come to a complete stop over time. As the hormonal shift occurs, we may also start noticing physical changes in our bodies.

Usually, a woman would know that they are approaching menopause when they start experiencing the symptoms, but if you need a doctor to confirm this, he or she may perform any of the following tests:

- Measure levels of follicle-stimulating hormone (FSH) and estradiol, which is a form of estrogen. FSH is a hormone that plays an important role in the functioning of the ovaries and testes in men. If your blood levels are consistently 30mlU/mL or higher, and when combined with no menses for 12 consecutive months, this could be confirmation that you are indeed in menopause.
- Another test is a diagnostic test called the Anti-Mullerian Hormone enzyme-linked immunosorbent assay (PicoAMH Elisa), which usually confirms menopause.

- One can also get over-the-counter (OTC) tests and saliva tests, but these are less reliable and can be pricey too.

If you go to a doctor, they can order other tests as well, and they will combine this with a look at your medical history to rule out the presence of any underlying conditions. These tests may include thyroid testing, liver function, blood lipid, testosterone, progesterone, prolactin, estradiol, and chorionic gonadotropin (hCG) tests, as well as kidney function tests.

## WHAT ARE THE SYMPTOMS OF MENOPAUSE?

The most commonly reported symptoms are irregular menses, periods that are heavier or lighter than usual, and what are referred to as *vasomotor* symptoms. Those are hot flashes, flushing, and night sweats. Research indicates that hot flashes can start around a year before menopause and could persist up to 20 years postmenopause, but on average, they last about five years (Koothirezhi & Ranganathan, 2021). This study also found that hot flashes affect approximately 70%–80% of those who are going through menopause.

Other symptoms of menopause that are not as well-known as those listed above are vaginal dryness, insomnia, depression, weight gain, anxiety, memory problems, concentration problems, reduced sexual libido, sore or tender breasts, headaches, racing heart, increased urination, urinary tract infections (UTIs), and many others (Huizen, 2023).

Some of the less noticeable symptoms that are, however, serious are loss of bone mineral density (BMD), which could lead to osteoporosis, raised cholesterol levels, and an increased risk of heart diseases and strokes (Office on Women's Health, 2019).

## WHAT HORMONES ARE INVOLVED DURING MENOPAUSE?

There are a few hormones involved in your menopause journey, but the main ones are estrogen, progesterone, and testosterone. Other hormones like FSH and luteinizing hormone (LH) also play a supportive role. Let's look at each of these hormones individually.

### Estrogen

Estrogen is one of the two main sex hormones, partnering with progesterone, and it is mainly produced in the ovaries, although small amounts of it are also produced in the adrenal glands.

There are three main types of estrogen: estrone (E1), estradiol (E2), and estriol (E3). During the childbearing years, a woman's body produces mainly estradiol. Estriol is the most common during pregnancy, and estrone is the only one produced after menopause.

Estrogen plays a key role in a woman's body from puberty on to help bring about physical changes and start the menstrual cycle. Its main function is to control the menstrual cycle, which makes it a key hormone for fertility and maintaining a pregnancy. Estrogen levels fluctuate throughout the month, peaking during the cycle and lowering during the actual period. During this time, estradiol will enable the development and release of the egg; in other words, it controls ovulation. It may surprise you to learn that estrogen is also involved in brain function, mood, bone health, and heart health. Previously, we mentioned the risk of increased cholesterol levels as a woman goes through menopause, mainly because estrogen is also responsible for regulating cholesterol levels.

**Estrogen During Menopause**

We know that estrogen levels decrease over time as one approaches menopause. Normal levels of estrogen vary from 45-854 pmol/L in premenopausal women. In menopausal women and beyond, these levels decrease to less than 100 pmol/L. Usually, the two hormones—estrogen and progesterone—balance each other, but as menopause approaches, estrogen levels start to fall, and one of the first signs that a woman is approaching menopause could be irregular periods.

**Estrogen and Bone Loss**

Estrogen plays a significant role in preventing the thinning and weakening of bones. When this happens, it could lead to osteoporosis. Women could lose up to a fifth of their bone mass when estrogen levels decrease (Forth, 2020). Your doctor might perform a test called bone densitometry, which is used to measure the amount of calcium in certain parts of your body. This test will confirm if you have osteoporosis or a condition called osteopenia. Osteopenia shows that your bone density is decreasing and is a precursor to osteoporosis. A diet rich in calcium and magnesium will be essential at this stage, and you may want to consider adding a vitamin D supplement and light exercise. Dr. Keay from Forth advises women to consider taking up weight training or incorporating exercises such as dancing and/or yoga to load the skeleton (Forth, 2020).

## Progesterone

Progesterone is a steroid hormone. It is produced by the body when you are ovulating, and its main function is to prepare your body for pregnancy. It does this by preparing the lining of the uterus, the endometrium, to receive a fertilized egg when there is a pregnancy. However, if there is no pregnancy, the endometrium will be shed as your period. Progesterone is initially produced by a temporary gland called the *corpus luteum* that develops after you ovulate, but later on, if a pregnancy occurs, its production shifts mainly to the placenta. Progesterone increases during pregnancy because its main role is to create a conducive environment for the egg first to be implanted and then to grow by thickening the endometrium. Its levels will continue to grow with each trimester of pregnancy, reaching its peak in the third trimester.

## Progesterone and Menopause

This hormone, however, declines as the woman approaches menopause.

As estrogen peaks during ovulation and progesterone assumes control in pregnancy, the balance between these hormones is disrupted as estrogen levels decline in the approach to peri-menopause. This can cause an imbalance that can show up as heavy periods. This is because one of the functions of progesterone is to regulate bleeding.

Another symptom of low levels of progesterone is vaginal dryness, and this is because progesterone thickens the mucus that is in the cervix, so less of it shows up as vaginal dryness.

Other functions of progesterone are: improving mood; supporting the function of the thyroid; and supporting lactation once a woman starts breastfeeding. From this, you can see that many symptoms of menopause are brought about by the declining levels of progesterone in the body, especially in an environment where estrogen is also declining since the two work in tandem.

**Testosterone**

Most people think that testosterone is only a male hormone, but this is not true. This hormone plays a significant role in a woman's body as well.

Testosterone is mainly produced in the ovaries and the adrenal glands, and it plays a number of roles: regulating the libido, arousal, and orgasm, as well as maintaining normal metabolic function, mood, cognitive function, and bone and muscle strength (British Menopause Society, 2022). The normal levels of testosterone that are produced in the bodies of young, healthy women are 100–400 mcg a day, which is three to four times higher than the amount of estrogen produced in their ovaries (British Menopause Society, 2022).

**Testosterone and Menopause**

Even though this hormone also decreases with age, the decrease is not as dramatic as that of estrogen and progesterone. In fact, levels of testosterone decrease by half between the ages of 20 and 40 (Forth, 2020). If you look at the role of this hormone as discussed in the above section, you will see that declining testosterone will show up as declining cognitive function, low libido, and mood swings, and it also, unfortunately, contributes to the risk of osteoporosis. Some women may also develop acne and facial hair during post-menopause, but this will be determined mainly by genetic factors.

All in all, you can see that the physical and psychological changes that a woman goes through during menopause are a result of the shifting landscape of hormones in their body. This also explains why hormone replacement therapy (HRT) is the main treatment offered when women are unable to cope with the symptoms.

## BEYOND HOT FLASHES: WHAT'S REALLY HAPPENING?

Usually, when you ask most people to list the symptoms of menopause, they talk about hot flashes, and this is because hot flashes are the most commonly talked-about symptoms. The danger in this is that it reduces menopause to just being about hot flashes when there are, in fact, many other symptoms that are just as serious, if not more so. I want to address those in this section.

### Irregular periods

This is one of the definite signs that you are nearing menopause. Over time, your period will completely stop, and after 12 months of not getting them, you can say you are now officially in menopause. We discussed how both estrogen and progesterone work in tandem during your menstrual cycle to regulate your period and that, as you approach menopause, the two hormones' levels start decreasing dramatically. When this happens, you start experiencing periods that are too heavy, too light, or less frequent.

### Brain Fog

Brain fog is one of the lesser-known symptoms of menopause. It wasn't until recently, when celebrities like Davina McCall started talking openly about the symptoms of menopause, that brain fog started receiving attention. Initially, people tended to reduce brain fog to minor annoyances, such as forgetting people's names, or you would often hear jokes about a woman going into the kitchen and forgetting what she was going to get there. But now we understand that brain fog is so much more serious than that, as it is now being labeled as "memory defectiveness," and some women report being scared that they may be experiencing an early onset of dementia when this happens.

We also know that brain fog is caused by declining hormone levels. While declining progesterone is known to cause sleep disturbances, mood swings, and brain fog, estrogen causes confusion, hot flashes, decreased energy, and brain fog (Simplyhealth, 2023).

Brain fog shows up in three ways: *forgetfulness, poor concentration, and poor information retention.* This not only impacts a woman's social life or relationships but their career life as well.

**Weight Gain and Slowed Metabolism**

It's estimated that menopausal women gain 1.5 lbs a year on average and that approximately 2/3 of women aged 40–60 are overweight (Ward Nutrition, 2020). Unfortunately, this weight gain also increases women's risk of other health conditions, such as heart diseases and certain cancers.

During menopause, when estrogen levels drop, the fat distribution changes, with the fat shifting from being stored in the hips to being stored around the belly. Also, as estrogen drops, proteins trigger the body's fat cells to store more fat and also slow down the metabolism of that fat (Santosa & Jensen, 2012). If you combine that with the fact that most women will tend to exercise less as they age, you will see that we have the perfect recipe for weight gain during this time.

**Anxiety, Depression, and Mood Swings**

Approximately 23% of women in peri- and postmenopause experience mood swings (North American Menopause Society,

2023). Research shows that fluctuations in estrogen can bring about changes to the brain and the nervous system and that these changes affect mood (Women's Health Research Institute, n.d.). This also affects sleep patterns, and as we all know, lack of sleep causes mood swings. As women face both physical and psychological changes, this affects their mood negatively and may increase their anxiety and depression as they struggle with their new identities. Another example is when a woman loses her sexual libido and how this may contribute to her being depressed, and the opposite can be true too—depression could cause a low libido.

**Sleep Disruptions and Insomnia**

As the hormones start fluctuating, this may disrupt your sleep patterns. According to Pacheco (2022), around 12% of women in general struggle with sleep, but that percentage increases sharply to 40% during perimenopause. Sleep problems worsen and continue right through postmenopause. Some of the problems with sleep that women report are sleep-disordered breathing, hot flashes or night sweats, and insomnia. Severe night sweats also cause insomnia, as women often struggle to fall back to sleep after experiencing them. Insomnia may cause other problems, such as impaired focus the next day, headaches, anxiousness, and irritability.

The Sleep Foundation reports that around 61% of post-menopausal women experience insomnia (Pacheco, 2022). Obstructive sleep apnea is also more common in post-menopausal women, and research indicates that this could be due to the reduced levels of progesterone. As if that wasn't enough, a woman's risk of sleep apnea increases by four percent each year of perimenopause (Mirer et al., 2017).

Declining estrogen also contributes a great deal to poor sleep patterns since estrogen also plays a significant role in the metabolism of serotonin. Serotonin is a neurotransmitter that plays a key role in regulating mood and sleep, among other body functions.

**Sexual Dysfunction and Lack of Desire**

Earlier, we mentioned vaginal dryness as one of the conditions caused by decreased levels of progesterone in a woman's body. Many women complain that sex hurts when this happens, and so they stop enjoying it. The North American Menopause Society (NAMS, 2023b) reports that between 17% and 45% of women experience painful sex.

Women also report experiencing a decrease in sexual libido during menopause, which causes marked personal distress around this condition. This condition is called hypoactive sexual desire disorder (HSDD). The results of a cross-sectional study done in the US on 2,000 women aged 30 to 70 showed that the number of those who reported this jumped from 26.7% in premenopause to 52.4% in postmenopausal women (West, 2008).

The decline in hormonal levels also causes the vaginal walls to become thinner, less flexible, dry, and fragile, a condition called vulvovaginal atrophy. Other women may experience a condition called atrophic vaginitis, where the vagina becomes inflamed, and when this happens, it becomes red and produces a discharge. Hormones are not the only cause of low libido, as this can also be triggered by stress, poor body image, depression, and frustration with how long it takes to reach orgasm (Levine, 2019).

## Brittle Nails and Hair Loss

During menopause, you may experience hair loss, a condition often referred to as female pattern hair loss in its extreme form (Levine, 2019). Some women also get brittle nails that may have ridges too. This is because of the declining levels of both estrogen and progesterone, whose other function is to contribute to healthy hair. We mentioned earlier that some women may start growing hair in unwanted places like the face due to the presence of the male sex hormone called androgen. Levine (2019) cites a study that showed that the blood that flows to the nail bed decreased by 30% in postmenopausal women compared to women in premenopause. Both hair and nails are affected by this because they are made of keratin, which, in turn, is affected by the decreased blood flow.

## Dry Skin and Other Skin Problems

Your skin may start getting dry, irritated, slack, and thin, and you may develop acne. You may start getting wounds that take a long time to heal and rashes. A woman may also get age spots due to sun damage. Age spots could also be a sign of a more serious problem, skin cancer, so it's best to have them checked.

You may develop jowls, and your skin could bruise easily. Again, estrogen is the culprit here, as it causes the skin to thin, leading it to bruise easily and suffer from all the above. Skin also loses collagen at this point, causing it to sag as it loses its firmness. This is because collagen provides our skin with structure. Research shows women's skin loses approximately 30% of its collagen in the first five years of being in menopause (American Academy of Dermatology Association, n.d.).

**Dry Mouth and Eyes**

Other symptoms of menopause are dry mouth and dry eyes, which could be a problem for those who wear contact lenses since the eyes lose their lubrication. Mouth dryness could lead to other problems, such as cavities, gingivitis, and periodontal disease. This, again, is caused by a decrease in estrogen; however, dry eyes are caused by a decrease in androgens. Research confirms that estrogen has the same effect in drying the mouth as it does in drying the vagina, as we discussed under sexual dysfunction. This is because it dries up the oral mucosa (Suri & Suri, 2014).

**Memory and Cognitive Function**

Earlier, we mentioned the example of walking into a room and forgetting why you went there in the first place as one of the common complaints by menopausal women. Some women report difficulties retrieving words during this time. The good news is that even though menopause affects cognitive function, the results do not seem to be permanent, as studied by Baylor

University (Sliwinski et al., 2014). These researchers also confirmed that even though declining estrogen is the main cause of this, other factors like sleep disruptions, night sweats, and depression also play a role in exacerbating the problem.

**Osteoporosis and Decreased Bone Health**

Healthy women build more bones than they lose up to the age of 30, but this changes after this age as bone loss starts occurring. This process is speeded up during menopause due to demineralization, resulting in osteoporosis in some (Cleveland Clinic, 2021a). This is mainly due to the declining estrogen levels since one of estrogen's key roles is to protect bone health.

## THE LESSER-KNOWN SYMPTOMS OF MENOPAUSE

In this section, we are going to discuss the lesser-known symptoms of menopause that most people don't even realize are related to menopause.

**Tingling in the Extremities**

Extremities may tingle, but this usually lasts for short periods of time and could be the reason most don't realize they are related to menopause. This is due to hormonal fluctuations, which affect the central nervous system.

**Cold Flushes**

These are thought to be caused by a change in the brain's ability to control body temperature (HCA Healthcare UK, 2023). They may happen spontaneously or immediately following a hot flash.

**Burning Mouth**

You may experience an uncomfortable sensation—tingling, tenderness, or burning—in your mouth, tongue, gums, or inside of your cheeks. Some women report that this could be severe, like burning your mouth with hot food, and this too is caused by decreasing estrogen levels. Remember that estrogen is responsible for supporting not only the structure of your bones and teeth but also the mucous membranes inside the mouth. Decreasing levels of estrogen impact oral health, as we discussed above, and this could result in a number of issues with the inside of your mouth, including bad breath.

**Change in the Sense of Smell**

You may notice that your sense of smell has changed; suddenly, you can't smell things as keenly as you used to. Another way your sense of smell is impacted could be when you notice that certain smells aren't pleasing to you anymore, and this is because the fluctuating hormones are affecting the pathways in the brain that control smell and taste. This may also cause a metallic taste in your mouth.

## Tinnitus or Impacted Hearing

This is a constant ringing or humming sound in your ears, and its severity may differ from one person to another. Your hearing could also become highly sensitive when you hear people chewing, breathing, and things like that. Tinnitus is a complex condition that affects the auditory pathways and may be made worse by other conditions such as depression, mood disorders, and stress. According to Newson Health (2023), depleting estrogen can negatively affect the auditory pathways and cause tinnitus. This is because there are estrogen receptors in the cells of our ears as well as along the auditory pathways.

## Dizziness or Vertigo

Since your inner ear is sensitive to estrogen, as explained above, when estrogen levels decrease, this could cause imbalances and impaired stability, which leaves you feeling dizzy. The other reason is that all three hormones—estrogen, progesterone, and testosterone—affect the widening and narrowing of your blood vessels, and when these hormones' levels start to decrease or fluctuate, this may leave you feeling light-headed or dizzy (Newson Health, 2023). Another contributor could be the fluctuating hormones affecting insulin production, causing instability in blood sugar levels (HCA Healthcare UK, 2023).

## Heartburn

Heartburn or acid reflux can leave an unpleasant taste in one's mouth, cause bad breath, and sometimes leave you feeling nauseous and bloated. Even though, in many cases, heartburn is caused by the type of food we eat, it can also be a symptom of perimenopause and menopause. This is because estrogen can change the amount of acid produced in the stomach. Cortisol, the stress hormone, can also affect digestion. A study done on 500 women showed that 42% of perimenopausal women and 47% of menopausal women experienced heartburn (Infantino, 2008).

## Itchy or Crawly Skin

You may start noticing that your skin feels dry and itchy at times. When estrogen levels drop, the skin becomes thinner, as we mentioned earlier, and as it loses its moisture, it becomes drier and itchy. Sebum, the natural skin lubricant, is affected by the depletion of estrogen, which contributes to the skin drying out.

Formication is another skin condition that occurs during menopause. It can be likened to the sensation of ants crawling on the skin.

## Breast Tenderness or Heaviness

Some women experience breast heaviness that is almost similar to what you'd experience when you are breastfeeding, and this condition is called mastalgia. This, too, is caused by estrogen fluctuations. The good news is that this gets better as menopause progresses. If, however, your breasts have puckered skin or if there is liquid coming out of your nipples, you should get that checked by a doctor, as it could be a sign of something more serious.

You may experience a loss of fullness of the breasts during this time as well.

**Body Odor**

Body odor may change during menopause, and there are three reasons why this happens:

- You may be sweating more, especially at night if you suffer from night sweats, and more so if you find that your antiperspirant is no longer as effective as it used to be. This could also be triggered by certain foods that you eat (Midlife Makeover, 2023).
- Some women start suffering from incontinence during this period, and this may be another cause for the strange odor.
- The third reason for this to happen could be due to the changing pH levels of your vagina because of the hormone fluctuations, resulting in a slightly different odor.

**Thinning Hair**

The fluctuations of hormones may cause your hair follicles to shrink, which will result in thinning hair.

**Heart Palpitations**

These may last for a couple of minutes or even a few seconds, and it's when you feel like your heart is beating more rapidly or in an irregular pattern than normal. They can happen concurrently with a dizzy spell, night sweats, or just randomly on their own. According to Newson Health (2023), the changing hormone levels affect the pathways in your heart through which the electrical impulses travel, thus causing the palpitations. On their own, heart palpitations are not serious, but you should definitely consult a doctor if they are accompanied by chest pains or shortness of breath or if they increase in severity and/or regularity.

Other symptoms that a woman might experience could be electric shocks, her voice changing, bloating episodes, or digestive problems, as well as the development of new allergies. It is very important to remember that no two women will go through or experience exactly the same or all of the symptoms we have discussed, so please do not be alarmed by the long list of symptoms covered here. This is just to make sure that we cover as many as possible, to help you recognize them should you experience one or a number of them.

## THE LINK BETWEEN BODY, MIND, AND SYMPTOMS

In this section, I want to talk about how stress exacerbates the symptoms of menopause.

Going through menopause on its own can be very stressful. Because you are experiencing both physical and psychological symptoms that are new to you, this can be scary and induce stress and anxiety. At the same time, stress can also create physical and psychological symptoms in your body, and now you find yourself caught in this never-ending loop. Furthermore, fluctuating hormones change the way we respond to stress, plunging us into depression and anxiety and leaving us feeling overwhelmed and isolated (Lee, 2019).

To understand this better, we need to look at the role of hormones again. Cortisol, which is the stress hormone, is produced in the adrenal glands. So is adrenaline. The two work in conjunction to produce what is commonly known as the "fight-or-flight" response to stressful situations. The adrenal glands also produce a bit of estrogen, as we mentioned earlier, but it's not their main function. When a woman goes into menopause, the adrenal glands will continue playing this role because estrogen and progesterone levels are depleting at this point. However, if you are experiencing stress, the adrenal glands will prioritize producing the stress hormones over the fertility hormones—simply because the body needs to be kept alive more than it needs to be kept fertile. Now, if a woman is facing chronic stress, the adrenal glands will eventually suffer from adrenal fatigue because they are constantly overworked and flooded with cortisol and adrenaline. When this happens, you may experience burnout, leading to other conditions, such as exhaustion, depression, insomnia, foggy brain, and even weight gain (Lee, 2019). Chronic stress also puts you at risk of more serious conditions like strokes, heart attacks, and diabetes.

## HOW DOES STRESS EXACERBATE THE SYMPTOMS?

**Hot Flashes**

Stress triggers hot flashes because it puts pressure on our nervous system. When this happens, the nervous system becomes "jumpy" and starts releasing adrenaline and histamine (Durward, 2019). These, in turn, cause hot flashes and/or night sweats.

**Mood Swings**

This one is very clear: If you are stressed by something happening externally—in your family, in your career, or other parts of your life—this will affect your mood, especially if you feel that you are unable to cope with whatever the issue is that's brought stress into your life.

**Weight Gain**

Weight gain is usually caused by declining estrogen levels, which cause a shift and redistribution in fat storage during menopause. This is the reason why many women gain undesirable belly fat at this stage. Gaining weight may also trigger stress and cause one to suffer from depression as they struggle to come to terms with the physical changes in their body. Stress may cause a woman to overeat as a source of comfort. Overeaters often indulge in sweet stuff, which leads to further weight gain. Stress may deplete the sodium levels in the body, and this triggers overeating since it creates food cravings. When one is depressed, their chances of working out are also slim, as their mood is impacted, and working out may be the last thing they want to do. All these factors interact with each other to create the perfect recipe for weight gain and depression.

## Insomnia

Menopause definitely impacts sleep. Women in this phase of life may struggle to fall asleep, and when they do, they may wake up in the middle of the night and struggle to fall back to sleep due to fluctuating estrogen levels. Also, if a woman is depressed and anxious due to the presence of other menopause symptoms, such as a lack of sexual desire, which impacts their relationship, this will impact their ability to fall asleep as well. Thirdly, for those who are also experiencing night sweats, waking up drenched in sweat is a major disturbance in one's sleep and will also negatively impact one's ability to fall back asleep.

## Digestive Problems

Stress affects one's digestive system. You may find that your digestive system is switching on and off throughout the day, resulting in indigestion, bloating, and constipation (Durward, 2019).

CONCLUSION

In this chapter, we have broken down what menopause is and discussed the accompanying symptoms in detail. Even though we have covered quite a list of symptoms here, the aim is not to scare you. As mentioned earlier, not *all* women will experience *all* of these symptoms, but this is just to give you the full spectrum of the symptoms to help you recognize them when you experience them. What we know for sure is that almost all of these symptoms are temporary, and even though the duration may vary from person to person, you will not have to deal with them for the rest of your life. So that's the first piece of good news.

The second piece is: In the introduction to this book, I mentioned the Radiant Shift Method (RSM), a method that will alter your perspective and enable you to view menopause in a new light. The RSM will help you reframe your experiences and help you see menopause not as an ending or a decline but as a vibrant transition into a new phase of life with its own strengths and potential. In other words, I'm inviting you, as you navigate these waters, to adopt an attitude of grace and power that will help you set the stage for a future filled with growth, connection, and radiant joy.

The last part of this chapter was dedicated to discussing stress and emotions, and so I want to invite you to dive with me into the subject of emotions in more detail in the next chapter.

# 3

# TIDES OF EMOTION

> *So many women I've talked to see menopause as an ending. But I've discovered this is your moment to reinvent yourself after years of focusing on the needs of everyone else. It's your opportunity to get clear about what matters to you and then pursue that with all of your energy, time, and talent.*

— OPRAH WINFREY

## FLUCTUATING HORMONES AND MOOD SWINGS

The role of hormones in the body can be summed up to these three things: "tell the body what to do, how to do it, and for how long" (Montare Behavioral Health, 2021). Since they are the chemical messengers passing communication from one cell to the next, when there is a hormonal imbalance, this manifests as certain symptoms or illnesses in the body.

When there are no hormonal imbalances in our bodies, with each of the hormones we have discussed in the previous chapter doing its job optimally, it promotes emotional well-being. In other words, estrogen will do what it's meant to do, which is to ensure that there is plenty of serotonin and dopamine produced in the body. These are the happy hormones. Testosterone will also do its job of making sure that there is enough dopamine activity. On the other hand, progesterone, working with the neurotransmitter GABA, will promote calmness and contentment. It will also make sure that there is plenty of glutamate, another neurotransmitter that promotes contentment and mental alertness. From this, you can see that everyone is happy when *everyone* is doing their job.

But what happens when there is an imbalance of hormones? A hormonal imbalance directly impacts the hormones, which then become dysregulated and, in turn, wreak havoc on our emotions. The result leaves us with feelings of anxiety, feeling low, and being demotivated. This could trigger negative or unhealthy behaviors such as overeating, avoiding exercise, alcohol abuse, and so on.

## ESTROGEN AND MOOD CHANGES

Estrogen plays a significant role when it comes to the emotional well-being of women, from their reproductive years all the way through to menopause. Firstly, it's involved in serotonin production, a neurotransmitter that regulates your mood. Fluctuating estrogen levels have also been associated with mood disorders that affect women only, such as premenstrual dysphoric disorder (PMDD), premenstrual syndrome (PMS), and postpartum depression (Hoffman, 2022). Estrogen clearly has anti-depressive effects on the body. High levels of it, however, aggravate feelings of tension or anxiety due to the imbalance that it causes (Herrera, 2019). You might find that women who have high levels of it in their bodies are prone to panic attacks and anxiety. The opposite is also true: Women with low levels of estrogen will be prone to episodes of depression. Studies show that around 18% of women suffer from depression at the beginning of perimenopause, the period when estrogen levels start declining, with this number going up to 38% at the end of this phase (Freeman, 2015). The good news is that depression rates fall after menopause and become almost similar to what we see in men.

## THE LINK BETWEEN ANXIETY AND PROGESTERONE

A recent study identified progesterone deficiency as a primary factor in anxiety patterns during midlife. In this study, cited by Herrera (2019), patients who had high levels of estrogen paired with low levels of progesterone exhibited extreme rage, followed by "a conciliatory, self-defeating demeanor". Progesterone seems to have a calming effect on the brain, with its deficiency manifesting in anxiety.

Progesterone may also have a balancing effect in cases where the body is producing excess adrenaline, helping to calm the mind down. Excessive adrenaline has a negative impact on the mind and could manifest as anger, depression, attention-deficit/hyperactivity disorder (ADHD), post-traumatic stress disorder (PTSD), addictions, and others. In fact, there is a growing interest and new research being done that focuses on the role of progesterone in treating other mental health conditions such as schizophrenia and bipolar disorders.

## CORTISOL AND MENTAL HEALTH

Cortisol is known as the stress hormone; however, it regulates other systems in the body, such as cognitive function, metabolism, and immune responses. We mentioned in the previous chapter how it works in tandem with adrenaline to induce a flight-or-flight response when facing what the body perceives as danger or stress. When you are under chronic stress, your body becomes flooded with cortisol, and too much of it is not good for you because it can trigger other health-related conditions such as anxiety and depression, sleep problems, and digestive problems, to name a few. During menopause, cortisol levels are naturally elevated, which gives your body the impression that it is under constant stress.

Progesterone helps to keep cortisol under check, but during menopause, when progesterone levels are also fluctuating and/or declining, this effect is compromised, leaving the body under stress. When this happens, it will trigger some of the menopause symptoms listed above, such as disrupted sleep, brain fog, fatigue, and anxiety, and affect your metabolism, which leads to weight gain and other symptoms. These, in turn, create more stress for you, which negatively impacts your mental health, placing you in this never-ending, vicious cycle.

## HOW PHYSICAL SYMPTOMS IMPACT MENTAL HEALTH

As a woman goes through physical changes in her body, this negatively impacts her mental health as well. Lack of sleep, often accompanied by night sweats, disrupts sleep, and less sleep impacts mood. So you may find yourself being irritable the next day, tired, or suffering from poor concentration and/or brain fog. Hot flashes can also trigger anxiety and depression as the woman struggles to deal with them.

In the previous chapter, we mentioned that some women experience painful sex due to a dry vagina and that this, too, is a result of declining estrogen levels. If this is you, this may cause you to lose interest in sex, which has a further negative impact on your mental health.

Weight gain is another trigger for depression, as a woman feels unable to control the steadily climbing pounds and the most annoying roll of fat around the waist. This, too, may trigger unhealthy behaviors like indulging in snacks as a way of comfort eating, which further exacerbates the problem.

Of the women who took the Kindra Menopause Symptoms Quiz, 42% reported feeling moody (KINDRA, 2017), and in other studies, women have listed being unable to sleep, feeling unusually irritable and anxious, and having panic attacks during this time.

EMOTIONAL FLUXES: BURDEN OR A JOURNEY TO
SELF-AWARENESS AND GROWTH?

Interviewed when she turned 50, Ms. Whoopi Goldberg said, *"All of a sudden, I don't mind saying to people, 'You know what? Get out of my life. You're not right for me. It's wonderful and liberating"* (McCaffrey, 2006).

How you experience menopause has a lot to do with how you approach this phase of life. Yes, the symptoms may be challenging, but they are temporary; it's a phase, which means it's not the rest of your life. A little shift in your perspective can help you view this as a new beginning instead of the end, and that will set you up for a rich and full experience of this stage. This could start with you not viewing it as a crisis, as in a "midlife crisis". Instead, you could choose to focus on the positive aspects of menopause, such as no more periods, becoming more in touch with your intuition, and finding "your voice," which means not being afraid to speak your mind and finding new ways of being intimate with your partner.

Dr. Trudy Smith, President of the South African Menopause Society (SAMS), advises women to view menopause as a journey that presents an opportunity for women to take stock of both their lives and lifestyles and make the necessary changes that will benefit their well-being and future (SAMS, 2019). Perhaps see this as a time of reflection and personal growth. By that, I mean that this could be the time that you spend asking yourself questions that would stimulate more growth on your part. I am talking about a different kind of growth—one that's not physical but one that helps you acquire more wisdom and personal fulfillment.

Some of the questions you can ask yourself during this time are, "Am I happy in my current relationships?" If not, "What can I change?" "Am I living a well-balanced life?" All of these will help you create a life that is fulfilling and joyful for you. During self-reflection, you may come to the realization that while you were chasing a career, you may have neglected your health, and now it's time to reclaim that aspect of your life. So you join a yoga or meditation class. Or maybe you never got the opportunity to travel and explore the world, so you revisit your bucket list and put that into action. You also get an opportunity to evaluate your friendships to see if these are the types of friendships that contribute to your well-being, and if not, there is no point in keeping them. If you were raising a family, you could have been so busy taking care of everyone else that you neglected yourself. Now is the time to make yourself a priority. Basically, menopause gives you an opportunity to recreate the life that you always wanted—you get a new lease on life.

There are certainly ways to transform your menopause experience and make it more enjoyable, and here are a few suggestions from the North American Menopause Society (NAMS, 2023a):

- Being mindful of your thoughts or watching your thoughts: It turns out that the absence of positive thoughts has more of a negative impact than the presence of negative thoughts on our health and well-being.

- Laughing more: Did you know that laughter has health benefits, including stimulating your immune system, enhancing your learning and memory, and helping you cope better with life stressors?
- Staying connected: Having social support is said to be the key to helping you live longer. Consider joining a support group.
- Staying in the moment: Staying in the present keeps you from worrying about the future, which creates unnecessary anxiety, or being fixated on the past, which may lead to regret.
- Making time for yourself: By incorporating exercise and self-care activities into your daily routine, you could reduce the amount of stress on your body and bring about dramatic changes to your health.

Other ways that you can take care of yourself during menopause are: practicing meditation, journaling, breathing exercises, and joining support groups for women who are in the same life stage. Let's talk about the benefits of each of these methods for a moment.

MEDITATION

Meditation helps you to focus on the present moment, helping to anchor yourself during emotional fluxes, and it enhances self-awareness. Practicing mindfulness is a way to bring us back into the present, and it's very much related to one or two of the above suggestions from the NAMS. When you're focusing on the present, you do not worry about the future or the past, which lessens your stress. So meditation helps you feel centered, and, according to psychologist Markesha Miller, when you're centered, "the world doesn't look so overwhelming" (Abramson, 2022). Research confirmed that meditation may be good for alleviating menopause symptoms, including fending off hot flashes (Manocha et al., 2007).

The great thing about meditation is that it can be done anywhere, and you don't need an expensive gym membership, just some quiet space. Here are some tips to help you incorporate meditation into your routine.

First of all, you may want to download an app. There are a few free meditation apps available online. Calm and Insight Timer are two of the most well-known, and they have free versions as well. You may also want to try out these meditation techniques:

**Body Scan Meditation**

This involves sitting down in a quiet place and performing a scan of your whole body, starting from the top of your head and focusing on each part of your body one by one to listen in for any pain, tension, pressure, temperature, or any other strange feeling until you get to the bottom of your feet. By focusing on your body, you help your mind slow down and remove the focus from anxious thoughts and external stimuli that could be the cause of your stress and tension.

**Sensory Grounding**

Focusing on your five senses is another way of removing the focus from anxious thoughts and grounding yourself in the present moment. You can do this by sitting down with your eyes closed and your hands on your lap facing up, then choosing to listen to the sounds around you, such as a car passing by, the coffee machine's gurgling sounds, and so on. This will definitely help you focus on the present moment. You can get up once you feel relaxed enough.

**Loving-kindness Meditation**

Being kind to yourself, also known as self-compassion, has been shown to improve your well-being and help manage stress (Abramson, 2022). How does one practice self-compassion meditation? Sit with your back against the wall and put your hand on your chest. Speak kind words to yourself, and you can do this out loud. You can also picture those who you know care about you saying these encouraging things to you.

**Bedtime Meditation**

Meditation helps you prepare your body and mind for sleep, thus reducing the likelihood of insomnia.

Lie down with your eyes closed and focus on your breathing, where you breathe in through your nose and out through your mouth. Then picture your breath going in through the nose and spreading out all through the inside of your body into the various parts—heart, lungs, hands, and feet. As you breathe out, imagine the air leaving your body and taking all the tension with it. So you have to imagine the in-breath coming in to energize your body and the out-breath sweeping out all the toxins and tension.

Hopefully, as you do this, you will start drifting off to sleep, which is the goal of this meditation exercise.

**Journaling**

Since menopause is not just a physical experience but an emotional one as well, you tend to feel a lot of emotions during this phase. What do you do with those emotions? Writing about one's feelings offers a form of emotional release, helping to clarify thoughts and process emotions. This is where journaling comes in handy. Some people see journaling as a way to show gratitude, ponder life, ease stress, or tap into their inner wisdom (Albarda, 2021). Here is a list of both mental health and personal development benefits that one can get from journaling, as suggested by *Midlife-A-Go-Go* (Albarda, 2021):

- It can help transform one's emotional well-being.
- It can help increase one's self-awareness.
- Journaling is great for setting and maintaining your goals.
- It can be a tool to examine life through one's own lens.
- It can help work through one's challenges.
- Use it to ask yourself probing questions so you have an opportunity to be honest with yourself.

- It can help you gain meaningful insights into yourself.
- It can help to heal from one's past.

There are no strict rules for doing this, but here are some guidelines that you should consider following.

**Consistency**

Consistency is key. Try to devote a specific time of the day to journaling, and that will help to keep you consistent. You may find that you write better at night just before going to bed, or you may be the type of person who prefers to do this first thing in the quiet of the morning. Let go of any judgment and just be authentically yourself, especially because your journal is for your eyes only.

**Allocate an Amount of Time**

Whether you give yourself 10 or 15 minutes to do it is entirely up to you. Some days, you will have a lot to write about, and some days, you won't, but setting an amount of time will help you protect it from interruptions. You may even consider putting your phone on flight mode during this time to avoid disturbances.

**What to Write About?**

The list of things you can write about is endless, but here are a few suggestions that you can use as prompts to help you get started.

- What would you say to your younger self—some piece of advice?
- What three things would you like to change about yourself?
- Where would you like to be three to five years from now?
- What are you grateful for today?
- What's missing from your life right now that you would like to change?
- Fondest memory of your childhood?
- Fondest memory of your adulthood?

## Breathing Exercises

Deep breathing or guided breathwork can calm the nervous system, reducing stress and emotional reactivity. Breathing exercises can help reduce stress, cool the body and mind, relieve an anxious mind, and offer stillness (Codrington, 2021). It offers other benefits too, such as anchoring you into the present and easing feelings of being overwhelmed. Here are three breathing techniques suggested by Kate Codrington:

## The Heat-Wave

Lay down on your back with your knees up and your feet on the ground. While resting your hands on your belly, soften your abdomen and prepare to take in deep breaths. Inhale through your nose as you allow your belly to rise, and exhale out of your mouth while letting the belly fall. Make a soothing sigh to calm your mind, and let go of the heat as you exhale. In other words, use this to go with the heat flash in a wave pattern when it comes.

Next, while resting one hand over your ribs and the other over your belly button, take a deep inhale, this time with a three-part breath. First, let the belly rise; next, feel the ribs expand; and finally, fill the lungs with air all the way to the chest. Exhaling slowly with a soft sigh out of your mouth releases the heat and/or stress. This should help calm the mind.

Try repeating this 8–10 times while slowing down the exhalation in each round. This will help calm your nervous system. Each time you do this, imagine this to be a wave of the hot flash rising from your belly and moving all the way through to the chest. If you like, you can visualize this wave in a certain color as it passes through you, or as light or heat. Practice doing this so that when a real heat flash comes, you can do this instead of tensing and/or panicking. This way, you can go with the flow when faced with a heat flash and allow the heat to flow through you and pass on. With time, you can do this automatically to calm yourself through the heat flash instead of trying to resist it.

**The Pursed Lips Breath**

As if mimicking the action of drinking through a straw, inhale with pursued lips. Stop and close your mouth when you get to the top of your breath, and then release the air by breathing out slowly through the nose. When you get to the top of your breath, try to swallow the air before you exhale. This swallowing will help to activate the vagus nerve, which controls the heart rate as one of its functions, and so this action can induce a calming effect.

## The Bee-Hive

With this breathing technique, we incorporate sound, which can stimulate the vagus nerve, thus producing a calming effect, as explained above. Inhaling softly through your nostrils, pause when you get to the top of your breath, and with a closed mouth, make a sound like that of a bumblebee as you exhale. Each time you get to the end of your exhale, pause before you start another breathing round. When you get to the end, sit for a minute and listen to the humming sounds' effect on your body.

## STRATEGIES FOR NAVIGATING EMOTIONAL CHANGES

On this journey, you will encounter circumstances that will trigger certain emotions in you. We all have things or situations that trigger us in one way or another. An emotional trigger can be a memory, an experience, or an event that triggers an emotional reaction from us, no matter what mood we were in previously. So what's the best thing to do when this happens?

See menopause as a growth opportunity, not just a challenge. There is a lot of truth in the saying, *"Your attitude determines your altitude,"* and we can apply it here as well. It also helps to have open communication with those close to you, so I encourage you to share your feelings with loved ones to gain mutual understanding.

Then, set boundaries. Identify your emotional triggers and establish personal and social limits to protect your mental health. Knowing your triggers and how to deal with them is the key to good mental health.

Raypole (2020) suggests listening to your body as a way to identify your triggers. Your body sends you "signals" when something is making you uncomfortable, such as sweaty palms, an upset tummy, a pounding heart, and/or shakiness or feeling dizzy when triggered. She suggests that when this happens, you take a step back and trace the roots of the trigger to understand it deeply. The next step is to own your feelings by choosing a different response to how they may have gone down in the past, because this allows you to take back control. Then, give yourself some space by moving away from the trigger and doing some breathing exercises to calm yourself down. When triggered by another person, it also helps to see things from their perspective, knowing that it may not be about you but what they are also going through at that moment that causes them to behave in a certain way. Once you have followed these steps, communicate your feelings with the said person in a calm and objective way to help them see how they have upset you. This should prevent a similar situation in the future.

The above suggestions, however, are there to help you deal with the situation as it happens, but you need strategies for the long term, and that's where the next set of suggestions comes in.

**Mindfulness Meditation**

We discussed some of the benefits of meditation in the section above, but essentially, we know that mindfulness helps you to be more aware of your emotions as they come up throughout your day. Research shows that mindfulness meditation might help to improve one's ability to process emotions and regulate them (Wu et al., 2019). You will benefit greatly, therefore, by adding mindfulness meditation to your toolbox.

**Identify Toxic Relationships**

You are not responsible for other people's behavior, but you have control over yourself and how you handle your triggers. If you have a friend who triggers you in some way or another, it is your responsibility to protect yourself from that, and one way you can do that is by removing yourself from the trigger. Consider stepping away from the friendship if the other person has no respect for your boundaries.

**Talking to a Professional**

Talking to a professional will offer you a safe, non-judgmental space to express your feelings and the opportunity to have someone else point out things that may be too close for you to see. A therapist can also give you communication tools to help you communicate your feelings better when talking to others, and they may provide guidance and support on your journey as you heal your triggers.

**Learning to Set Boundaries**

According to Pattemore (2021), boundaries are a form of self-care because understanding how to set and maintain them can help you avoid feelings of resentment, anger, and disappointment that often build up when you are pushed beyond your limits. She further explains that boundaries help you establish what behaviors you can expect from others and what they can expect from you.

Boundaries can be as strict or as loose as you want them to be, depending on the situation or the environment. For instance, you may have stricter boundaries at work than at home. Pattermore lists five types of boundaries: physical, sexual, financial, emotional, and intellectual. She explains that physical boundaries may be easier to spot when they are being crossed, but you have to rely on your own internal signals when emotional or psychological boundaries are being crossed.

How, then, do we set healthy boundaries? Here are some guidelines to help you:

**What Are the Reasons for Your Boundaries?**

The first step, which is also very important, is to take some time to reflect on the reasons why you need to set boundaries. Is it because of the way people treat you or how something makes you feel? How will setting boundaries help you achieve emotional well-being? These questions should give you some indication of whether you need to set boundaries in your interactions with others or not.

**Start Slowly**

Start by establishing a few boundaries and seeing how that makes you feel. After that, you can continue adding more. Setting too many boundaries at once may be overwhelming for you. Remember, too, that you can always tweak them as you go, depending on how you feel.

**Set Boundaries Early**

Setting boundaries earlier in your relationship means you don't have to wait until lines are crossed to do so. This sets the foundation for a healthy relationship, as it lets everyone know where they stand and what will be tolerated versus what won't. That way, you can avoid confusion, hurt, and resentment later on.

**Be Consistent With Your Boundaries**

It would be very hard and confusing for others to know how to deal with you and respect your boundaries if you were not consistent with them. Being consistent helps reinforce your beliefs and original thresholds and ensures that those lines are clearly established.

**The Importance of Carving Out Time for Yourself**

Spending time with yourself may be a great way of taking care of yourself, and there are a myriad of things that you can do during that alone time. You could go for long walks, take yourself out on a date, get some spa treatments, or simply stay in and read a book. Protecting that time by letting your loved ones know that it's your alone time is a form of creating boundaries, and it will definitely boost your well-being.

**Consider Adding Extra Personal Boundaries**

You should not be afraid to add your own extra boundaries, even if you are in a workplace where boundaries already exist. A study done in Australia showed that employees who had personal boundaries in the workplace felt more empowered (Hornung, 2019).

**Setting Boundaries on Social Media**

These days, it is very easy for boundaries to be crossed, especially on social media, where friends and family can share your photos without your permission. You have every right to enforce boundaries online just as much as you do in real life, but you will have to communicate those clearly to your loved ones.

**Always Communicate Clearly When Lines Are Crossed**

Communicate your boundaries clearly without being confrontational.

## Love Yourself by Engaging in Activities That Make You Happy

Participating in activities that spark your joy is a form of self-love. These could be activities like dancing, getting a massage, doing yoga, or whatever the activity is—by doing this, you are sending a message to yourself that lets you know that you are worth it and deserving of nice things.

## Gain a Healthy Perspective of Your Boundaries

Going overboard with setting boundaries can be detrimental to your mental health as much as not having any would be, warns Dr. Quinn-Cirrillo, a UK-based psychologist (Pattemore, 2021). She advises that we should have a healthy level of thinking about boundaries and be careful of overthinking them or having our lives dictated by them.

Here is a final word on boundaries: When you expect others to respect your boundaries, it's important that you also return the favor by respecting theirs, so get to know theirs too by asking. For instance, you could ask a friend if it's okay to call them after a certain time before you do so. When you show that you respect other people's boundaries, they will respect yours too.

STAYING ACTIVE

Exercise is great for releasing those mood-boosting endorphins and improving our overall quality of life. There are many other benefits that staying active brings into our lives, and I'm going to discuss a few of them here.

**Preventing Weight Gain**

In earlier sections, we mentioned the effect that fluctuating levels of both estrogen and progesterone have on our metabolism, which results in changes in fat distribution, causing, among other things, abdominal fat. During menopause, women also lose muscle mass, which slows down the rate at which our bodies burn calories. Adding lifestyle and genetic factors to the mix creates a perfect recipe for weight gain. Exercise has been shown through science to help prevent weight gain and muscle loss (Mayo Clinic, 2023).

**Decreasing Risk to Other Health Conditions**

In relation to the above point, weight gain puts you at risk of other health conditions such as cardiovascular diseases (CVDs), certain cancers like endometrial and breast cancer, type-2 diabetes, and strokes (Better Health Channel, 2022). Exercise, therefore, lessens this risk for you.

## Improving Bone Strength

Once a woman reaches the age of 30, her bone strength starts decreasing, and this is exacerbated by declining estrogen levels during perimenopause. Reduced bone density increases your chances of getting osteoporosis or brittle bones. Exercise is a great way to prevent this from happening because it improves your bone strength, the strength of your muscles, and your balance. This in turn reduces your risk of falling (Silver, 2019).

## Improving Mood

Exercise improves your mood because it triggers the release of endorphins, the "feel good" hormones (Rodriguez, 2023). This endorphin release, which occurs an hour after exercise, relieves pain and stress, and it boosts your sense of well-being—what is called the "runner's high", says Dr. Paulvin, who is a regenerative medicine doctor in New York.

Exercise also stimulates the release of serotonin, another mood hormone, and this is great for us menopausal women as our moods are often negatively impacted by menopause symptoms.

## Reducing Stress

Exercise not only helps to improve mood, but it also relieves stress and lowers the symptoms of anxiety and depression (Mayo Clinic Staff, 2020). It also reduces the release of cortisol, the stress hormone, thus lessening the harmful effects of stress on your body. This relief from stress helps us women cope better with menopause symptoms, which ultimately improves our quality of life.

There is a body of research that shows that exercise lowers the risk of depression because of its positive effects on brain function. It is responsible for the creation of new nerve pathways that improve cognitive function, which ultimately decreases the symptoms of depression (Powers et al., 2015).

**Improving Sleep**

Exercise reduces the incidence of insomnia (Wild, 2023), and when you sleep better, you feel better and more energized the next day, which means you are not stressed by a lack of sleep. There is a study that showed that those who participated in 150 minutes of moderate-high-intensity training a week were able to significantly reduce the severity of insomnia symptoms and instead elevate their mood (Hartescu et al., 2015).

## WHICH EXERCISES ARE BEST IN MENOPAUSE?

**Strength Training**

Strength training seems to be the best type of exercise simply because it tops the charts when it comes to strengthening your muscles and bones. Improving your muscle tone is great for weight loss, and improving your bone strength is great for preventing osteoporosis, both major concerns for menopausal women. Strength training also improves your metabolic health, which means a lower risk of CVDs and diabetes (Wild, 2023).

This type of training, also called resistance training, is also good for speeding up one's metabolism and burning fat. You don't even need to join an expensive gym to be able to do this, as long as you have some resistance bands, some free weights, or kettlebells at home. You can also find many exercise classes or accounts to follow on YouTube, and as soon as you find one you like, it will be easier to stick with it. You can also do yoga and/or pilates online. Of course, if you have access to a gym, you can use the weight machines and the free weights and/or join a weight training class.

**Balance and Mobility**

Maintaining balance reduces your risk of experiencing falls as you grow older since balance can be decreased by the loss of muscle mass during menopause (Wild, 2023). The other benefit of doing balance and mobility training is that it helps improve your body-mind connection, which means it can help lower your stress levels. Some of the exercises you can do to improve your balance and mobility are tai chi, pilates, and yoga.

**Cardio**

Cardio activities include walking, jogging, dancing, cycling, swimming, high-intensity interval training (HIIT), and running. Cardio is great for improving heart health because it improves the efficiency with which your heart pumps blood. The health of your blood vessels and lungs is also improved through doing cardio exercises, and this is especially important for menopausal women, whose risk for heart health is greater after menopause (Wild, 2023). Cardio is not only good for your heart, but it also has other health benefits, such as improving the quality of your sleep, boosting your mood, and increasing your energy levels.

Incorporating at least 150 minutes of exercise into your weekly routine has great health benefits, and it only works out to about 30 minutes of exercise, five times a week.

## SLEEP TIPS WHEN YOU ARE IN MENOPAUSE

The Sleep Foundation reveals that sleep problems increase dramatically from about 12% of women, in general, having sleep problems to 40% of women in their 40s and 50s, which further increases to 50% of menopausal women experiencing this problem (Wright, 2023).

The most common sleep problems that have been identified in menopause are insomnia, hot flashes, obstructive sleep apnea (OSA), restless leg syndrome (RLS), and anxiety and depression, which contribute to an inability to fall asleep. The fluctuating levels of both estrogen and progesterone contribute to this since they impact the body's ability to produce serotonin.

Wright (2023) suggests the following tips to help improve sleep:

- Have a regular sleep schedule and follow it. This means going to bed at the same time every night and getting up at the same time, including the weekends.
- Avoid taking naps, especially in the late afternoon, since this may affect your ability to fall asleep.
- Have a bedtime routine. This could be anything from listening to relaxing music to reading, meditating, etc. Try to set aside at least 30 minutes for your nighttime routine.
- Avoid or reduce screen time before bed. The light from devices like the TV, phones, and tablets interferes with the sleep cycle and could mess up your circadian clock.
- Keep your bedroom at a comfortable temperature that is not too hot or cold.
- Exercise at regular times each day, but not close to bedtime. Exercising for 150 minutes per week significantly reduces hot flashes by 18%, sleep problems by 21.5%, and joint discomfort by 48% (Javadivala et al., 2020).
- Avoid eating large meals close to bedtime. Digestion slows down later in the day, and your body has to work harder to do this, preventing restful sleep.
- Avoid caffeine late in the day. Many people know the effects of caffeine as a stimulant, and with coffee having a half-life of five hours, it can take that long for it to keep you awake (Wright, 2023).

- Avoid alcohol before bed. Alcohol disrupts the quality of your sleep, despite its sedative effects. It can also make you feel tired the next day.
- Use relaxation techniques. Relaxing helps improve the functioning of the autonomous nervous system, which controls digestion, heart rate, and blood pressure. It also assists the parasympathetic nervous system, which slows down the body's activities and ultimately relaxes us.

### SEEK PROFESSIONAL HELP

Consider therapy if emotions become too challenging. Therapy has been proven to be a very powerful treatment for depression (WebMD, n.d.-b). Other benefits of therapy include

- helping you change the behaviors that are holding you back and develop fresh insights.
- helping you cope with menopause symptoms
- teaching you how to handle certain emotions such as anger, disappointments, and so on.
- evaluating your thinking patterns that may be affecting how you feel
- helping you heal from the pain or disappointments of the past
- helping ease or manage stress

## CONCLUSION

In this chapter, we discussed the emotional changes that take place during menopause, the hormones that play a role in triggering certain emotions, and suggested various tools that you can use to help you manage or deal with those emotions when they surface.

We also spoke at length about the importance of creating boundaries, the benefits of exercise, and how to get good-quality sleep. I hope that all these tools help you get a better handle on your emotional state. I'm very excited about the next chapter, which will see us getting more in touch with our intimate feelings as we delve deeper into the nuances of sexuality during menopause.

# 4

# A NEW DAWN OF INTIMACY

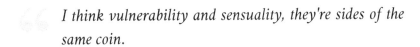

*I think vulnerability and sensuality, they're sides of the same coin.*

— RENE MARIE

## THE ASSUMPTION OF "DIMINISHED" WOMANHOOD

Throughout history, many societies have seen fertility as the primary role of women, often tying it to their societal values. This can be traced back to Biblical and ancient times when it was "shameful" for a woman to not bear a child, and this is unfortunately still pervasive in today's society. Phrases like "biological clock" perpetuate the idea that there's a ticking time limit on a woman's fertility and, by extension, her significance. The pressure is on so much that you may see it in the number of women who are unable to conceive a child naturally and often seek assisted reproduction procedures like in-vitro fertilization. We see this in the booming medical tourism industry as people travel to other countries where these medical procedures are more affordable in an effort to do whatever it takes to satisfy this "insatiable" longing to bear a child.

Womanhood isn't just about childbirth; it encompasses a range of experiences and roles across a lifetime. Older women have far more wisdom, and we need to recognize the value that comes with age. Menopause can open doors to new experiences, roles, and avenues of self-discovery that were previously overshadowed by reproductive responsibilities.

Then there is the issue of the woman's youth being treated like a commodity, or her most valuable asset, but one that has a clock on it, soon to expire. It makes us women feel like we come with an expiration date. This obsession with women's youth is further promoted by pop culture and the media. What's with magazines featuring topics like "You can still look sexy at 40" and advertisers pushing anti-wrinkle creams and serums everywhere you look? What about Botox, breast lifts, and tummy tucks? All of these are there to help us fight the "devastating" effects of aging. They say the beauty industry is a billion-dollar industry, and there are no surprises there.

And, as Bennett (2014) puts it so eloquently in her piece *Stop Telling Women that Their Most Valuable Asset is Their Youth,* "the youthfulness we are chasing is not about biology and is not solvable by science," but rather a cultural message that we need to stop listening to.

## REDEFINING SENSUALITY AND INTIMACY

### How Menopause Affects Sexual Desire

Over 1/3 of women who are in perimenopause or post-menopause report experiencing sexual problems that range from loss of desire for sex to challenges with getting orgasms (Johns Hopkins Medicine, n.d.). However, not all women go through this, as there have been some women reporting an improved sexual drive post-menopause (WebMD Editorial Contributors, n.d.). Those who report this name their newfound freedom of being empty nesters and not being concerned about falling pregnant as contributing factors to this increased desire. Normally, sex drive wanes with age, although reports show that women are twice or even three times more likely than men to be affected by this (The North American Menopause Society, n.d.-a).

### What is sexual desire?

The NAMS describes it as "interest in sex and in being sexual". They explain that sexual desire has three components: drive, beliefs, and motivations.

### The Three Components of Sexual Desire

- Desire is the biological aspect or component that shows up as fantasies, thoughts, erotic attraction, genital tingling, or wanting to engage in sexual activity. We also call it the libido.

- Beliefs, values, and expectations around sexual activity, on the other hand, are affected by your own attitudes toward sex, and they, in turn, are affected by cultural and religious beliefs, those closest to you, as well as the media (The North American Menopause Society, n.d.-a). So, those who have positive beliefs or attitudes toward sex generally have a greater desire for sex.

- Motivation speaks to your willingness to engage in sex with a particular person at a particular time. This is the most complex component simply because it is greatly affected by emotions and interpersonal factors and is more recently being viewed by experts as the most important component of the three.

### How Does Menopause Affect Sex Drive?

During menopause, you may notice that you are no longer easily aroused and may even find that you have become less sensitive to touch, so your interest in sex may decrease. With the fluctuating hormonal levels, specifically estrogen, and testosterone, you can expect that one of the areas of your life that will get impacted is your sex drive. Naturally, sex drive varies from person to person and day to day depending on our stress levels and other activities, but declining estrogen and testosterone have a major impact. On top of that, a drop in estrogen levels decreases the supply of blood to a woman's vagina, which results in less lubrication for the vagina, making it feel dry and less stretchy.

There are other factors that negatively impact a woman's desire for sex during menopause, and they include lack of sleep, night sweats, hot flashes, depression and anxiety, bladder control issues, stress, and medications.

**Dryness, Discomfort, or Pain**

Some women also experience vaginal dryness, which causes discomfort during sex and pain for some. The vaginal walls also become less stretchy, contributing to the discomfort experienced during sex. Also, according to Kraft (n.d.) of Johns Hopkins, as we age, it takes a bit longer for blood to fill our genitals, which reduces the sensitivity, and we, therefore, take longer to reach orgasm. Throw in other health problems that a woman may be experiencing at that time, which may make her feel depleted of energy, as well as body image issues. All these things reduce a woman's desire for sex. HRT offers relief for those who suffer from vaginal dryness, and this comes in a vaginal ring, a cream, or a pessary, should you want to use it.

**Does Menopause Lower Sex Drive in All Women?**

The short answer is no. There are reports of postmenopausal women who report increased sex drive. Researchers think this could be due to the fact that these women don't have to worry about things like childbearing responsibilities and pregnancies and often suffer less from anxiety.

**Desire Usually (But Not Always) Wanes With Age**

We know that desire wanes with age in both males and females, though it affects more women than men, as we mentioned previously. For women, this usually starts around their 40s, but it differs from woman to woman. The symptoms of menopause also contribute to this decreased desire; as you can imagine, when a woman is dealing with hot flashes, night sweats, anxiety, and depression, the last thing on her mind is sex. Doctors also think that low levels of testosterone could have something to do with reduced desire; however, scientific studies haven't proven this. If you suffer from a recurring and persistent lack of desire, you may be diagnosed with a condition called "hypoactive sexual desire disorder", a condition that is very common among women.

**Sensual vs Sexual**

Is there a difference between the two, and if so, what is it? Secrets Boutiques (n.d.) describes sensuality as "the ability to fully experience and appreciate life through our five senses". Sexuality, on the other hand, has a lot to do with the physical intimacy between two consenting adults. Sexuality is more about expressing our sexual desires, fantasies, and preferences in a physical and emotional manner (Shaw, n.d.). The two are often used together or interchangeably because being physically intimate or being sexual involves the senses, and that makes it sensual. However, the opposite is not always true because you can be sensual without engaging in sexual activity.

Dr. Rosara Torrisi, a practicing sex therapist, describes sensuality as the basis on which we experience our bodies, the bodies of others, and the world we are surrounded by (Shaw, n.d.). Sensuality can be a way to create a connection with others but also with ourselves, for instance, when you take a nice, long, warm bath, get a massage, or eat a nice meal. In this way, we can view sensuality as an essential component of, or another form of, self-care, intimacy, or self-awareness.

**The Role of the Five Senses**

If you think about how we use our senses on a daily basis, it is easy to see the role they play in helping us connect with the world sensually. Your sense of taste, for instance, when you are eating ice cream or a delicious meal, and your sense of hearing when you listen to beautiful music as you are winding down at the end of the day. What about touching as you rub your skin with lotion or getting a caress from another person? Imagine, too, when you see the sky lit with vibrant colors as you watch the day slowly turn into evening. The smell of coffee in the morning or your favorite perfume brings your sense of smell to life. These are all examples of the various ways in which we engage our senses that help us enjoy a more sensual life.

**Emotional Connection: The Significance of Intimacy in Sensuality**

Emotional connection, or intimacy, is the foundation of any successful relationship, but we have to allow ourselves to be vulnerable with our partners in the process of forming that connection. Being vulnerable means opening yourself up to share your deepest feelings, insecurities, and desires with your partner in a safe, non-judgmental space. Once we have created a comfortable environment, we are free to explore our sensuality, which will deepen our pleasure in profound ways, heighten our experiences, and help us bond with our partners. This makes sensuality a very powerful aspect of our relationships.

**Mindfulness and Presence: The Importance of Being in the Moment**

Mindfulness is about being present and engaged completely at that moment, and this happens both on an emotional and physical level. It's about noticing everything that's happening with your senses and enjoying being in your body. There are a number of activities that you can engage in to enjoy being fully in the moment. Think about dancing. As you sway and twirl around the room, you are fully in the moment. What about cooking your delicious meal and tasting and savoring the flavors as they come together in the masterpiece that you are creating?

**Ways to Experience Sensuality**

You experience sensuality through your five senses, as I've already mentioned above. Explore touch by giving yourself a massage, using a tennis ball, or your hands. How about rolling on the grass? Or feeling the warmth of the sun on your face and body?

What about smell? Visit a candle store and walk around, smelling the different candle scents. You can get the same effect by visiting a perfume store. Or by smelling freshly baked bread.

With regard to taste, what about trying a foreign dish? Or making a really delicious dessert for yourself?

When it comes to sight, have you tried watching a lava lamp in action? Or lighting a fire or a candle and watching it burn.

To indulge my sense of hearing, I prefer listening to some lo-fi music while I work. For you, it might be the sound of a baby laughing or a waterfall tumbling.

## EMBRACING A DIFFERENT KIND OF SEXY

So far, we've been talking about how to be sexy and/or sensual, but now I want to shift our focus to talk about other qualities that make a woman attractive regardless of her age. In fact, these qualities redefine *attractiveness*, and like fine wine, they get better with age.

**Style**

Having a sense of style will always be attractive. Please understand that style is not what's trending, and so it doesn't come and go.

## Confidence

Confident women don't seek approval from others or need attention from others in the room. Someone once said, "Confidence isn't walking into a room and hoping they like you; it's knowing you're going to be fine even if they don't".

## Originality

This one speaks for itself; it's about being yourself and not trying to be anybody else.

## Class

Being classy has nothing to do with which wine you drink or which restaurants you eat at; it's about how you conduct yourself. It's definitely *not* about being a snob.

## Wittiness

A person who can make you laugh is generally attractive, because who doesn't want to be around them?

## Loyalty

Loyalty is attractive. Period. After all is said and done, you want someone who's got your back, so loyal people are keepers.

### Smarts

Like loyalty, intelligence is always going to be attractive, and it doesn't have to come in the form of someone with a degree from Harvard. Street smarts will see you through some situations, and you'll know it when you have it.

### Honesty

No one wants a liar. Period. An honest woman is one you can trust even in the dodgiest of circumstances, and I think everyone finds that attractive.

### Charismatic

This is about being charming, and it's a quality that draws or attracts people toward you and keeps them wanting more of you.

There are many other ways to boost your self-confidence and embrace body positivity, such as using daily affirmations if you believe in their power. I know people who swear that their lives changed when they started using affirmations. You can find examples of affirmations for menopausal women online.

Also, choose to engage with media that celebrates women of all ages, stages, and body types. Avoid content that perpetuates unrealistic beauty standards. We all know what happens when we compare ourselves to those Instagram models with impossible beauty standards.

**Style Tips**

Rediscover your personal style by experimenting with clothing and makeup that make you feel confident and authentic. The focus isn't on trying to look as young as possible. It is about aging well. Remember these words from Coco Chanel: *"Nothing makes a woman look so old as desperately trying to look young"* (QuoteFancy, n.d.)?

Choose clothing that enhances your good parts, and as Gessica Marmotta, personal stylist, says, look at color, fabric, fit, and cut, and own the fact that your body may never return to what it was in the past (Marmotta, 2022). For more styling tips, check out Gessica's LinkedIn page.

**Skin Care**

When it comes to makeup and skincare, each woman will have different needs that they want to address, so you will have to choose accordingly. Some women may have age or sun spots, dry skin, skin that bruises easily, jowls or wrinkles, acne or pimpled skin, skin rash, or wounds that take forever to heal.

Some tips for taking care of your skin:

- Keep it hydrated by using a moisturizer. Moisturizers that contain glycerin, hyaluronic acid, and peptides can help improve your skin's elasticity and firmness.
- Drink your water, as this helps with hydrating the skin.

- Use sunscreen to protect you from sun damage. Get sunscreen with an SPF of at least 30, and wear it even on cloudy days.
- Retinol, which is a vitamin A derivative, boosts the production of collagen. This reduces wrinkles and fine lines and will improve your skin's texture.
- Get plenty of sleep. Poor sleep produces dark circles, fine lines, and dry skin.
- Add anti-oxidants. Anti-oxidants fight the free radicals that are responsible for premature aging.
- Avoid harsh products. Ask for a sample to test at home before you buy a full product if you are not sure how it's going to treat your skin. The worst mistake would be to buy a product that will strip your face of its natural oils or cause irritations.
- When it comes to makeup, remember that less is more. Jenny Patinkin, a makeup artist, warns us against using too much concealer because it can look dry and cakey on mature skin. It can also settle into fine lines and wrinkles (Julian, 2023). It's also best to choose hydrating concealers and foundations and to moisturize your skin well before applying makeup products.

## CONCLUSION

In this chapter, we explored various ways to feel confident and sexy in your own skin. We started by discussing ways to improve intimacy in your partnership that don't necessarily involve sex but engage our five senses. We then ended the chapter by sharing tips to boost your confidence by incorporating other qualities that never go out of style, improving your skincare, and sharing some style tips.

The next chapter delves into the subject of treatment for menopause symptoms, and we present both medical and holistic approaches so you can be well-informed as you decide what's best for you.

# MAKE A DIFFERENCE WITH YOUR REVIEW

*Change is the only constant in life.*

— HERACLITUS

**"Menopause and Beyond"** has been a journey of self-discovery and empowerment. As we close this chapter, *think about the big idea in this book*: Menopause doesn't mean a woman's light is going away—it's actually making her shine even brighter.

My mission is to make "Menopause and Beyond" accessible to all. That's where you come in. Most people judge a book by its cover and reviews. So, on behalf of a struggling woman navigating menopause, please help by leaving a review.

Your review takes less than 60 seconds but can change another woman's life forever. It could help one more small business provide for their community, one more entrepreneur support their family, or one more client transform their life.

To make a real impact: Scan the QR code below.

If you're the kind of person who finds joy in helping a faceless friend, welcome to our club. Your support means the world.

I'm thrilled to share upcoming chapters filled with tactics, lessons, and strategies that will help you navigate this stage of life with even more confidence.

Thank you sincerely,
Kate Hartwell

# BRIDGING WISDOM

*A positive attitude gives you power over your circumstances instead of your circumstances having power over you.*

— JOYCE MEYER

## HORMONE REPLACEMENT THERAPY (HRT)

In the first chapter, we discussed how one of the main functions of estrogen is to control the menstrual cycle, making it a key hormone in fertility and maintaining a pregnancy. So, this hormone is at its peak functioning during your reproductive years. When you enter perimenopause, estrogen levels start fluctuating. Progesterone works with estrogen; however, its main function is to support the health of the uterus so that a pregnancy may occur. Both hormones will start fluctuating and declining in menopause, but when this happens, they upset the functioning of other bodily processes. As a woman who is in perimenopause, you will start experiencing menopause symptoms when this happens.

Estrogen has other functions too, such as contributing to the heart, brain, and blood vessels health, but another one of its important functions is its contribution to healthy bones. So a woman who is in menopause may also develop osteoporosis if her bone health is compromised.

## THE BENEFITS OF HRT

In its simplest form, HRT replenishes the hormones that are decreasing as you enter menopause, which helps lessen the menopause symptoms. HRT simply means taking estrogen, and for those who still have a uterus, you would take progesterone (progestin) as well. So you would often hear of two types of HRT: estrogen-only therapy (ET), when you take estrogen only, and combined estrogen plus progestogen therapy (EPT), when you take a combination of estrogen and progesterone. This is to protect those women who still have a uterus from endometrial (uterine) cancer if they take estrogen only. For those who are on ET, estrogen may be taken as a low dose in a pill or patch every day but can also be prescribed as a gel, cream, spray, or vaginal ring. It's advisable to take the lowest dose possible that can relieve the symptoms.

The symptoms that HRT alleviates are hot flashes, night sweats, vaginal dryness, anxiety, and low mood and sleep problems (NHS, 2023). Relief from symptoms is usually felt within a few days of starting HRT. HRT can also help with protection against osteoporosis since it replenishes the estrogen that is necessary for bone health. This is especially recommended for those whose periods stopped before they reached age 45 or if they went into early menopause. A large study that is mentioned in Cedars Sinai (n.d.) was done on 25,000 women aged 50–79 in post-menopause and showed that HRT significantly reduced the risk of bone fractures. HRT can also help improve muscle strength, which is usually affected by age.

Why is it recommended that those who still have their uterus take EPT instead of ET? When you are still in your reproductive years, you shed the endometrium lining every time you have your period. When this is no longer happening, taking estrogen alone can cause an overgrowth of cells in your uterus, which could lead to endometrial cancer. Progesterone reduces the risk of this happening by thinning out the endometrium.

Those who had their uterus removed (hysterectomy) obviously don't need this type of protection and can therefore take ET. There are benefits to this too, because estrogen alone has fewer health risks over the long term. Vaginal estrogen, available in tablet, pessary, vaginal ring, cream, or gel form, helps to ease the condition of a dry vagina. Since it is taken locally, very little of it gets into the rest of the body, so it's not necessary for it to come as an EPT combination to protect women against endometrial cancer. In other words, it's safe to use as ET.

There are other health benefits of taking HRT that have been reported by women, and these are:

- reduced risk of diabetes
- decreased risk of colon cancer
- less
- some improvement in the occurrence of joint pains
- decreased number of deaths in women who take it in their 50s
- improvements in mood and general mental well-being

As much as these are great benefits, which is certainly a relief to know, we do have to talk about the risks associated with taking HRT.

## THE RISKS OF TAKING HRT

These are some of the well-known risks of taking HRT:

- greater risk of blood clots
- a greater risk of dementia in cases where HRT was started after midlife. However, when started during midlife, it's been shown to decrease the risk of dementia or Alzheimer's disease
- increased risk of gallbladder or gallstones
- increased risk of getting breast cancer, especially when taking it for a longer time
- reported cases of endometrial cancer if taken by those who still have a uterus and without combining it with progesterone, as discussed in the above section

## What is the Connection Between HRT and Heart Disease?

Maybe you are concerned because you have heard that there is a connection. The connection between the two is still a subject of inquiry, and the data is mixed right now, but what is coming out strongly is that it is all time-dependent, with less risk demonstrated for those who initiate HRT within ten years of menopause versus those who initiate it at a later stage (Hodis & Mack, 2022).

## What About Breast Cancer?

Data shows that HRT can slightly increase the risk of breast cancer, so it is not recommended for those who have already had breast cancer. The risk seems to be greater with longer-term use of HRT and age (NHS, 2023). The risk is also lower for those who take ET. It is, therefore, advisable to take the lowest dose of HRT as much as possible and not take it for longer than you actually need to alleviate the symptoms of menopause.

## Risk of Strokes and Blood Clots

HRT use has been associated with an increased risk of strokes and blood clots, although the risk is low for those who are under 60 (Cedars Sinai, n.d.). The NHS (2023) also reports that the risk for strokes and blood clots is higher for those who take it systemically, i.e., pills, than for those who take it locally (patches, gel, sprays). The level of risk also depends on your medical history and the type of hormones you take. I highly advise that you seek the counsel of your doctor, who will take all of these factors into consideration before he makes a recommendation, as this will be different from one woman to the next.

## WHO SHOULD NOT TAKE HRT?

HRT is not recommended for these women:

- if you have had breast or endometrial cancer
- if you have abnormal vaginal bleeding
- if you have liver disease
- if you have a history of blood clots or are at risk
- if there is a history of strokes, CVDs, or increased risk of such
- if you suspect that you may be pregnant

## WHAT ARE THE SIDE EFFECTS OF HRT?

Some of the most reported side effects of HRT are:

- monthly bleeding for those who take EPT
- irregular spotting
- mood swings
- tenderness of breasts

The less common side effects include headaches, fluid retention, increased breast density, which could be a challenge when doing mammograms, skin discolorations, and skin irritations for those who take their HRT via a patch.

The Cleveland Clinic (2021b) reports that these are usually mild and don't require you to change anything; however, if you feel that they are unbearable, you should speak to your clinician about adjusting your dosage.

Now that we have covered the basics of HRT, how it works, and the benefits and risks that it comes with, I would like to move toward clearing out some of the misconceptions and myths that surround HRT.

## HRT MYTHS

- HRT will delay menopause. HRT will not delay menopause, but it will help ease the symptoms that accompany it. It's possible that those who believe or perpetuate this myth reached that conclusion based on the occurrence of certain side effects that we discussed in the earlier section, where HRT sometimes causes bleeding and other conditions that make a woman seem like they are not in menopause.
- HRT is for menopause symptoms only. This stems from the belief that HRT is for women only, which is not true. Men who suffer from low testosterone also take HRT to address that condition.
- Only one type of HRT exists. We already spoke about the different types: ET and EPT, and these are prescribed after taking into consideration a woman's medical history. HRT also comes in two modes of delivery: systemic (tablets or injections) and locally

administered (patch, gel, vaginal ring, pessary, or cream).

- HRT is associated with heart attacks among menopausal women. This belief came about after the Women's Health Initiative (WHI) study, which enrolled women who were over 60 years old and received EPT. A follow-up study showed that these women were already at increased risk of heart attacks. After this, a recommendation was made that women initiate HRT within 10 years of menopause, before 60, because age plays a role in increasing the risk of heart attacks (Hodis & Mack, 2022).

- HRT causes breast cancer. Improper hormone replacement can wreak havoc on your body, especially if you have an underlying condition. So HRT is not recommended for women who have had cancer, and that's also the reason why ET is only recommended for women who have had their uterus removed.

- HRT causes blood clots. Clinical evidence shows that this risk is very low. It is estimated that out of 1,000 women who take HRT over seven years, only less than two might get a blood clot (Hormone Health, 2018).

- Calcium and vitamin D are better than HRT for protection against fractures. This is not true. Research has proven that HRT protects against bone fractures and osteoporosis because it helps increase bone density. Vitamin D and calcium, on the other hand, haven't been scientifically proven to have the same effect.

- Natural treatments work better than HRT. HRT has been scientifically proven to effectively relieve the symptoms of menopause, and we don't know if this is true for natural treatments since they haven't been scientifically tested.

- HRT should not be started too young. For women who go into early menopause and for those who have had hysterectomies, HRT can help replace those hormones that have a protective function against heart diseases and osteoporosis, so it's actually quite beneficial.
- HRT will cause weight gain. On the contrary, because HRT helps balance the hormones, it may give you a better handle on your weight. Combined with a healthy diet and regular exercise, you have no reason to fear that you might gain weight from HRT.
- It's best to wait until your symptoms are severe before you start HRT. This is not true, as we have already discussed the importance and benefit of starting HRT within the first 10 years of menopause.
- You can't take HRT for a period longer than five years. Obviously, it's best to take HRT for a short period, but a woman should take it for as long as she needs it, preferably at the lowest dose possible.

## WHAT ABOUT THE RESEARCH THAT SHOWED INCREASED RISK?

Newer research shows that the WHI study that showed a correlation between HRT and breast cancer, blood clots, and heart attacks was flawed. Two main things have been identified that were wrong with it: the type of HRT used and the age of the study participants. According to Dr. Klaiber, an endocrinologist from Massachusetts, we could have seen a different result had the study clinicians used a different regimen—estrogen-only instead of a combination pill (NBC News, 2005). The researchers thought it would be easier for women in the study to take a combined pill instead of having to remember to only take progesterone on a cycle of 10–12 days a month.

The second flaw was the age of the enrolled study participants, whose average age was 62.7. This age group is already at a higher risk of CVDs, so we don't get a realistic picture when we look at the data since some of them would have already been presenting with underlying conditions. Dr. Klaiber further explains that the risk for women in their 80s is 12 times higher for CVDs than it is for those in their 50s.

The last word I wish to say on this is that since no two women will go through the same experiences as far as their menopause is concerned, and with everyone having a different medical history, a proper medical consultation before you start taking HRT is a necessity to determine the best course and dosage for you.

HOLISTIC ALTERNATIVES

Now I know that not everybody is a fan of medical interventions, so I'd like us to turn our attention to holistic alternatives as an option to present a complete picture of what's available for women to choose from or what other women are using out there.

## Plant Estrogens

Also called phytoestrogens, these types of estrogens occur naturally in food. Isoflavones and lignans are the two types of plant estrogens that are well-known and are currently under study. The main sources of isoflavones are soybeans, chickpeas, and lentils, as well as other legumes. Lignans, on the other hand, are found mostly in whole grains, flaxseeds, and certain fruits and vegetables.

As pointed out, these phytoestrogens are currently being studied for their effectiveness in alleviating the symptoms of menopause, but some women have reported their benefits. Some report that flaxseeds and flaxseed oil help relieve night sweats. Sage, which is thought to mimic the effects of estrogen due to some of its compounds, has also been reported to help lessen menopause symptoms. This herb, however, should be avoided by those who are allergic to it or those with high blood pressure or epilepsy.

## Bio-Identical Hormones

Although these come from plant sources, the hormones in them are chemically identical to the hormones made by your body. Some bio-identical hormones are Food and Drug Administration (FDA)-approved, though many other products are mixed by pharmacists that fall under this label but haven't been approved by the FDA. Unfortunately, there is no scientific evidence that these are as effective or better than traditional HRT or that they carry less risk.

**Black Cohosh**

This is another popular supplement among those who report that it helps them manage vasomotor symptoms like hot flashes, but the data to support this claim is still inconclusive at the moment. A few studies have shown that, when compared to a placebo, it seems to have an effect, but others do not show this benefit (WebMD, n.d.-a). Those with liver problems and those with a history of breast cancer are warned to stay away from this supplement.

**Dong Quai**

This is an herb that has been used extensively in China among women to treat their ailments, but research has found no evidence that it helps. Some have warned that it might increase the risk of cancer when taken over a long period of time, so use with caution or, rather, speak to your health adviser before use.

**Maca Root**

This herb has been shown to offer a number of benefits, such as helping lower the effects of stress and aging. It does this by decreasing cortisol levels. It has also been linked to a reduction in low energy, hot flashes, and restlessness. It can also improve libido and prevent weight gain (Axe, 2023).

## Yoga

The main benefit of yoga that we know of is that the balancing exercises may help strengthen your bones and muscles, which will improve your coordination. This has the added benefit of preventing falls and, ultimately, fractures. Other than that, yoga hasn't been shown to improve the symptoms of menopause.

## Acupuncture

There is little evidence that this treatment may help ease menopause symptoms like hot flashes, but beyond that, there are no other known benefits in relation to menopause. Not much research has been done in this area.

## Hypnosis

There is some research that was done by the National Center for Complementary and Integrative Health that showed hypnotherapy may reduce hot flashes and improve sleep, thus helping reduce interference with daily life (Mayo Clinic, 2017).

## Adaptogen Herbs

Under this umbrella, we include medicinal mushrooms, ashwagandha, rhodiola, and holy basil. These herbs have been shown to have a number of health benefits, including improvement of thyroid function, decreasing depression and anxiety, stabilizing blood sugar and insulin levels, a reduction in the degeneration of brain cells, and improved cholesterol levels (Axe, 2023).

**Evening Primrose**

This is one of the most popular treatments for menopausal symptoms. Evening primrose is thought to help manage symptoms of menopause because it contains two types of omega-6 fatty acids: linoleic and y-linoleic acids, which increase the production of prostaglandins, which are hormone-like substances. Evening primrose is reported to help aid with the reduction of night sweats, hot flashes, sleeping problems, mood disturbances, and vaginal dryness, although the National Institute for Health (NIH) has said there isn't enough scientific evidence to support these claims. The only study that showed an improvement in the intensity of hot flashes enrolled women 45–59 years old and compared evening primrose to a placebo (Farzaneh et al., 2013). This study, however, didn't show an improvement in the frequency or duration of hot flashes.

To end this section, I want to say that it is obvious that both modern medicine and holistic approaches have something to offer women in alleviating their symptoms. Modern medicine can address certain symptoms directly, while traditional remedies might help manage broader, holistic aspects of well-being. Instead of choosing to go one route only, you could perhaps decide to combine therapies in order to reap the benefits of both. A combination allows for treatments tailored to individual needs. For instance, you might use HRT for severe symptoms but employ yoga for stress management. This is just one example, and as already mentioned, it will depend on your individual needs, as no two women will have the same.

## THE POWER OF MINDSET IN MANAGING SYMPTOMS

We all know the importance of mindset in shaping how we experience life. This is why you often hear sayings like "mind over matter," the one I mentioned earlier, "your attitude determines your altitude," and other similar sayings. Basically, what this means is that two people can go through the same experience but react to it in very different ways, and when this happens, the outcomes will be different too. It is the same with menopause. How you perceive it—whether you see it as a threat or as a stage of natural transition—can influence the severity with which you experience the symptoms.

Our mindset is often shaped by our past experiences and beliefs. Though we may not be able to go back and change our past experiences, there is still an opportunity to change our beliefs and the mindset that was created out of them. It's important to understand your own mindset so that you can see the impact that it has on your life. Do you have a fixed or a growth mindset? Hampton (2022) cites a study that demonstrated that after a single 30-minute session on a growth personality mindset, teenagers displayed higher levels of internal control as well as an improvement in their ability to cope with stress.

**So, what's the difference between growth and a fixed mindset?**

When you have a growth mindset, you subscribe to the school of thought that says your abilities can be developed by working hard. Those who have this mindset always work hard to improve and learn new strategies to improve their skills, personality, character, and intelligence. Those with a fixed mindset, on the other hand, believe that personality, intelligence, and character are fixed and can't be changed. Having this type of mindset can be a roadblock to your growth and to helping you achieve your goals and the life that you desire. So by having a growth mindset, or you can even call it an open mindset, you will be able to open yourself up to new ways of thinking and new ways of perceiving life, which will help you embrace every experience and see it as an opportunity for growth.

Approaching menopause with a mindset of acceptance and seeing it as a rite of passage can potentially mitigate stress and the intensity of some symptoms.

To conclude, in this chapter, we discussed ways to alleviate the symptoms of menopause by choosing between HRT and traditional or holistic remedies, though I invited you to consider the benefits of combining both types in order to reap the benefits of both. I ended the chapter by talking about mindset and the role that it plays in how you approach and experience menopause, as, in my humble opinion, it doesn't matter what intervention you choose; as long as your mindset is not right, it will undermine the whole experience. This will cause you to go through menopause as a stressed and depressed individual.

Since nobody wants to go through it in that state of mind, I have dedicated Chapter 6 to discussing strategies for how to attain a radiant life by making certain lifestyle changes.

# A RADIANT LIFE

*Take care of your body. It's the only place you have to live.*

— JIM ROHN

## HOW DOES LIFESTYLE IMPACT MENOPAUSE?

A person's manner of living, which is usually made up of their habits, moral standards, interests, attitude, economic standards, and consumption, is what makes up their lifestyle. Your lifestyle can be healthy or unhealthy depending on these factors, and this will directly impact your overall well-being. If your lifestyle is unhealthy, you will be at risk of many health issues, including metabolic disorders, CVDs, bone and joint issues, obesity, hypertension, and many others (Oswal, 2022). Likewise, if you maintain a healthy lifestyle based on eating a healthy diet, exercising regularly, and not indulging in any destructive habits, you will prevent many lifestyle diseases.

There are many examples of how lifestyle can impact your menopause experience. For instance, the Health Site (2016) cites a study that showed that a sedentary lifestyle worsened menopause symptoms in over 6,000 Hispanic women aged 40–59. This study linked a sedentary lifestyle to anxiety, depression, obesity, and insomnia. When compared to their active counterparts, these women were significantly worse off when it came to their experiences of menopause symptoms.

Other factors that have been identified as contributing to the worsening of symptoms are poor diet, too much alcohol, not getting enough sleep, low intake of water, poor exposure to natural light, and not taking preventative measures against one's mental and physical health. Basically, what this means is that the choices you make daily, from the foods you consume to the amount of sleep you obtain, can directly influence the severity and frequency of menopausal symptoms. Let's look at each of these factors and see how they impact our health.

**Poor Diet**

The effects of a poor diet on our health is a subject that has been studied extensively. So why is it that many people still eat poorly and risk their health? Oswal (2022) puts it down to lack of planning. Because we live such a fast-paced life, most people don't have the time to prepare healthy meals. It's always easier to grab a muffin on your way to work than to have a properly cooked breakfast. When you feel your energy dipping during the course of the day, you could be tempted to just grab a chocolate bar or a pack of crisps. She further explains that these habits sneak up on us, and before we know it, our waistline is growing.

It's also very important to take a good look at the types of foods that you include in your diet. When you eat a lot of spicy food, this could trigger your hot flashes and/or night sweats.

Your diet can impact not just your health but your energy levels as well. When you think of some of the diseases that a poor diet places you at risk of, such as diabetes, CVDs, strokes, and some cancers, it gives you a real wake-up call as to the importance of a healthy diet for your well-being.

**Too Much Alcohol**

According to Dr. Kling of the Mayo Clinic, using alcohol during menopause can make the symptoms worse. She warns us that the two can be a dangerous mix. Alcohol can exacerbate vasomotor symptoms, that is, hot flashes and night sweats (Hames, 2023). Dr. Kling also warns that while many people think a glass of wine in the evening will help them unwind and get a good night's sleep, it actually does the opposite because it disrupts the quality of our sleep. Her advice is to stay away from alcohol, especially the closer you get to bedtime. Alcohol is also associated with a high risk of breast cancer, weight gain, and other poor health outcomes. Maybe it's time to rethink your favorite drink or at least cut down on the amount you consume.

**Low Water Intake**

Your body gets dehydrated when you don't drink enough water, and generally, the recommendation for adults is 6–8 glasses a day. What happens when our bodies are dehydrated? You may experience frequent headaches, a dry mouth and bad breath, urinary tract infections (UTIs), kidney stones, feel dizzy or tired all the time, get constipated, and suffer from dull skin and hair (Oswal, 2022).

**Lack of Sleep**

The Mayo Clinic recommends that adults should get about 6–8 hours of sleep per night to be well-rested and focused the next day (Olson, 2023). However, as you get older, your sleep time shortens. You take longer to fall asleep, you wake up a number of times during the night, and you wake up early. The quality of sleep we get is compromised by stress, screen time, and having to deal with things like night sweats, etc. Unfortunately, lack of sleep also puts us at risk of various diseases like strokes, CVDs, diabetes, obesity, depression, etc. This happens because the body doesn't get enough time to repair its immune system and produce cytokines that fight illnesses. When we don't get enough quality sleep, we experience shortened concentration spans, loss of short-term memory, feel dull and drowsy the next day, and may even feel antisocial.

## Lack of Exercise

Data from Australia shows that between 2014 and 2015, almost half (45%) of adults aged 18–64 and 59% of those aged 65 and above were not living an active lifestyle (Australian Institute of Health & Welfare, 2016).

We have mentioned the importance of exercise a number of times in this book already, but I will mention it here again because it speaks to the subject of lifestyle, and since we are discussing the impact of our lifestyle on how we experience menopause, we have to revisit the subject. The main benefit of exercise is how it helps to keep the extra pounds at bay, and since weight gain is one of the symptoms of menopause, there is no question that an active lifestyle will be one of the weapons you use to fight the symptoms. Other benefits of exercise are to improve brain health, strengthen your bones and muscles, and lower exposure to some diseases. For those who do strength or weight training, there is an added benefit in that exercise increases bone density, which, as we know, reduces the risk of osteoporosis (Mayo Clinic, 2023a).

## Poor Preventive Monitoring of Physical and Mental Health

Health screenings are essential for early detection of underlying health issues, so doing them once or twice a year as part of your lifestyle is a preventative measure against many health issues. The health issues it could help you detect early are cancers, diabetes, depression, anxiety, CVDs, and others.

## Not Enough Exposure to Sunlight and Fresh Air

Spending too much time indoors could lead to feelings of loneliness, depression, stress, and a fluctuating mood (Oswal, 2022). This could be triggered by low serotonin levels. Remember, serotonin is the hormone that's responsible for regulating mood, sleep, and sexual desire, all of which are negatively affected during menopause. So, just by not spending time outdoors, you could exacerbate your experience of menopause symptoms. Other than boosting our mental health, sunlight also offers us a number of health benefits, such as producing vitamin D, reducing blood pressure, improving bone health, and preventing other diseases.

When it comes to fresh air, not getting enough of it has been linked to various health conditions such as high blood pressure, compromised immunity, obesity, and a negative impact on digestion.

## The Four Major Lifestyle Diseases

The four non-communicable diseases (NCDs)—diabetes, certain types of cancer, strokes, and CVDs—are all lifestyle diseases. They are called lifestyle diseases because they are essentially a result of one's lifestyle. There are four behavioral factors that place us at risk of these diseases: smoking, alcohol abuse, lack of exercise, and an unhealthy diet. For instance, a smoker may get lung cancer due to their smoking history. When it comes to CVDs and strokes, a number of behavioral factors place us at risk, such as poor eating habits, a lack of exercise, smoking, and alcohol abuse.

The good thing about behavioral factors is that they can all be changed, and when you adopt healthier behaviors, you address or prevent the majority of these lifestyle diseases. Menopause provides an opportune moment to assess your current lifestyle habits and make necessary adjustments to optimize your well-being during this phase. Take a closer look at your own lifestyle to see if there are any areas where you might need to make changes, and who knows? Just by making a few modifications, you may see an improvement in your general well-being and get some relief from some of your menopause symptoms.

## MENOPAUSE AND WEIGHT GAIN

As you grow older, it becomes increasingly challenging to maintain a healthy weight. Most weight gain happens around perimenopause, where you start to notice, among other things, a roll of fat developing around your waistline. Genetic factors also play a role, so if you had parents who carried weight in the abdomen, chances are you will too (Mayo Clinic, 2023b). So does lifestyle, as we discussed in the section above. This weight gain, unfortunately, places you at risk of other diseases like CVDs, breathing problems, and type-2 diabetes.

**What Is the Effect of Menopause on Weight?**

Some of the changes that your body goes through during menopause directly lead to weight gain. A few factors that contribute to this weight gain are fluctuating hormones, lack of sleep, loss of muscle mass, and increased insulin resistance. I'm going to briefly talk about each one individually.

## Hormone Fluctuations

Fluctuating levels of estrogen and progesterone will cause a shift in the distribution of fat as well as in the body's ability to burn fat, thus contributing to weight gain (Grantham & Henneberg, 2014). When this happens, it also places you at risk of metabolic diseases, CVDs, and type-2 diabetes.

## Lack of Sleep

There is research that shows that poor sleep contributes to weight gain (El Khoudary et al., 2019). This could also be due to the fact that your body doesn't get enough "downtime" to perform all the processes including properly digesting food.

## Insulin Resistance

As women, when we age, we become insulin-resistant, which makes it more challenging to lose weight (Mumusoglu & Yildiz, 2019).

## Losing muscle mass

A number of things contribute to this, and these include age, hormonal fluctuations, and less physical activity. Losing muscle mass slows down the rate at which the body burns calories, making it harder to lose weight.

**Importance of a Calorie Deficit**

The formula for weight loss is to burn more calories than the calories you consume. This is how you create a calorie deficit. Science shows, however, that as women age, they start burning fewer calories when they are at rest during menopause and postmenopause. The solution to this is not to reduce your calorie intake even more when you are trying to lose weight because your body will react by slowing down its metabolic rate as it adapts to this. This will not make you lose any weight, so my advice is to not be tempted to go on those crazy diets. Doing that would make matters worse too, because this negatively impacts your muscle mass (Weiss et al., 2017). Not only that but reducing your calorie intake also contributes to bone loss, further placing you at risk of osteoporosis.

## DIET PLANS THAT WORK WELL DURING MENOPAUSE

There are healthier diets that have been proven to be safer for menopausal women, which could help address the problems identified above. Some of these diet plans that work well during menopause are low-carb diets, the Mediterranean diet, and vegan or vegetarian diets. I'm going to talk about each one of these.

## The Mediterranean Diet

This diet has been consistently rated in the top 5 of all diets for good reasons. Well-known for its great health benefits, such as reducing the risk of heart disease and other chronic diseases, assisting with weight loss, and improving health, this diet has been extensively studied (Romagnolo & Selmin, 2017). One of these studies was done on Spanish women and showed that the diet reduced the risk of obesity by 30% in perimenopausal and postmenopausal women (Sayón-Orea et al., 2015).

The Mediterranean diet is mostly plant-based, meaning it consists mainly of legumes, vegetables, whole grains, fruits, and nuts, with olive oil as the main oil used. On this diet, you can also eat moderate amounts of dairy and small amounts of poultry, eggs, and meat.

The other great benefit of this diet is that it is pretty flexible, even allowing an occasional glass of wine, and no food groups are totally off-limits.

## A Low-carb Diet

Research shows that a low-carb diet is great for weight loss and decreasing abdominal fat (Goss et al., 2014). There aren't many low-carb diet studies that have enrolled menopausal women exclusively, but Thompson et al. (2015) found that postmenopausal women who were on a low-carb diet lost 27.5% of their body fat and 3.5 inches (9.9 kg) of their waist circumference. The paleo diet performed better at helping postmenopausal women lose abdominal fat and weight after two years when compared to a low-fat diet (Mellberg et al., 2014). The paleo diet draws 30% of its calories from carbs, so it's a low-carb diet.

**Vegan or Vegetarian Diets**

Both vegan and vegetarian diets are showing promise in helping women lose weight. Postmenopausal women who were randomly assigned to either a vegan diet or a National Cholesterol Education Program (NCEP) diet lost more weight at both Year 1 and Year 2 of follow-up (Turner-McGrievy et al., 2007).

These diets also seem to help alleviate vasomotor symptoms, as shown in a survey done in 2018, compared to omnivore diets. Including dairy and eggs, thus making it a vegetarian diet rather than a strictly vegan diet, could have more benefits for older women, according to the results of a study by Mahon et al. (2007).

## BEST TYPES OF EXERCISE FOR WEIGHT LOSS

Remember the formula for weight loss, *"more calories burned than calories consumed"*? Well, that's where exercise comes in, because exercise will help you burn all those calories that you're taking in through your diet. We already discussed the importance of exercise in different sections above and the importance of incorporating at least 150 minutes of moderate exercise into your weekly schedule.

Exercise has many health benefits that include weight reduction, mood improvement, and protecting your bones and muscles. Weight or resistance training has specifically been proven to increase lean muscle mass (Lera Orsatti et al., 2014). We know that lean muscle mass declines with age, so weight training should be in your arsenal for fighting a decline in health at this age. With resistance training, if you want to fight abdominal fat, research shows that the more training you do, the more benefit you will see.

Research has also shown that aerobic or cardio training is also good for weight loss for menopausal women and that it helps with abdominal fat reduction as well while preserving muscle (Earnest et al., 2013). I would, therefore, recommend that you combine the two to benefit from both. Combining the two will also keep you from getting bored with having the same routine all the time.

## LIFESTYLE CHANGES THAT PROMOTE WEIGHT LOSS DURING MENOPAUSE

Fixing your diet and incorporating exercise into your routine may be two of the best things you can do for yourself during menopause to fight weight gain, but there are other lifestyle tweaks you can add that would promote weight loss as well. Sleep is one of those. We have mentioned sleep before and the importance of getting at least six hours of good-quality sleep every day. Menopause symptoms make it harder to get quality sleep because some of them wake you up several times at night.

To make matters worse, research shows that those who get fewer hours of sleep have higher levels of ghrelin, the hunger hormone, and lower levels of leptin, the satiety hormone (Bonanno et al., 2019). You can clearly see what the impact of this would be on your waistline.

Other things you can do to improve your wellness that could also help with weight management are exploring the benefits of psychotherapy, acupuncture, and other stress-relieving methods.

Cognitive behavioral therapy (CBT) has been shown to help reduce insomnia. A study done on a group of postmenopausal women who received CBT over a six-month period showed increased sleep duration (Drake et al., 2018).

Acupuncture may be able to increase estrogen levels and promote better sleep (Avis et al., 2016). Acupuncture was also shown to reduce hot flash episodes by 36.7% in another study cited by Spritzler (2023).

It's also crucial to find ways to manage stress, especially if you suffer from chronic stress. Stress elevates the cortisol levels in your body, which puts you at risk of other health conditions and is associated with abdominal fat (Jackson et al., 2017). Incorporate stress-reduction activities like yoga into your weekly routine.

## DIET TIPS THAT WORK

The following tips have helped people lose weight at any age, including menopause:

- Load up on protein. Protein has been shown to increase satiety and metabolic rate and to reduce muscle loss in those who are trying to lose weight (Rains et al., 2015).
- Including dairy might help you lose fat and retain muscle, just like protein.
- Incorporating foods that are high in soluble fiber will increase your insulin sensitivity, help with weight loss, and reduce appetite.
- Through a review of studies, it has been shown that green tea contains both caffeine and another compound called epigallocatechin gallate (EGCG), which speeds up the fat-burning process (Vázquez Cisneros et al., 2017). Try to drink green tea as often as you can.
- The benefits of mindful eating should not be undermined, as this has been proven to help you develop a healthy relationship with food and reduce stress, so you eat less (Warren et al., 2017).

**Nourishing the Body**

While weight gain during menopause is a commonly discussed concern, it's essential to understand that nourishment goes beyond the scale. It shouldn't just be about managing weight; it's about embracing a holistic approach that prioritizes both physical health and emotional well-being. Here, we are going to discuss the relationship between our diet and mental health.

So, we know that the foods we consume can have direct impacts on our mood, thanks to the gut-brain axis, and I want to spend some time talking about this connection here. This connection is commonly referred to as the mind-gut connection. The connection between the two is so strong that the gut is now being referred to as the "second brain". The two are connected physically and biochemically. Before we explore that further, let's think of some examples of what happens when we eat certain foods. Sugar comes to mind as a good example. Sugar causes a temporary spike in your "feel-good" hormone, dopamine. This is when we experience what is called the "sugar rush", but as we all know, it's temporary, and soon after that, you come crashing down. Nutrient-dense food, on the other hand, stabilizes your mood and improves your ability to focus. Basically, what this tells us is that the food we eat affects the gut, and the gut responds by impacting or influencing our brains so that we feel certain emotions.

Nutritional deficiencies can exacerbate mood swings and fatigue, which are common in menopause. If you suffer from chronic stress, this can also alter the gut microbiota, which will further increase inflammation and make you susceptible to mood disorders. Furthermore, studies show that imbalances in the gut bacteria have the ability to impair certain cognitive functions like learning, memory, and attention (Northeast Digestive, 2023).

Now, let's explore the science around this connection a bit more.

## The Nervous System and the Vagus Nerve

There are 100 billion neurons in the human brain and about 500 million in the gut, and these neurons are connected via the super highway of the nervous system. One of the biggest nerves in the nervous system is the vagus nerve, and it works by sending signals both ways. Several studies have been done to investigate the role of the vagus nerve, and in mice, it was shown that although feeding them a probiotic decreased the amount of stress hormone in their blood, cutting their vagus nerve undermined this effect (Bravo et al., 2011). A study on humans showed that those with Crohn's disease and irritable bowel syndrome (IBS) had a decreased vagal tone, meaning the function of their vagus nerve was reduced (Pellissier et al., 2014).

The function of the vagus nerve is so significant that damage to it could lead to a condition called gastroparesis, a condition where food does not move into the intestines (Cleveland Clinic, 2022).

## The Role of Neurotransmitters

Neurotransmitters are the chemicals that also connect the gut to the brain. The neurotransmitters that are produced in your brain are responsible for mood, like serotonin, which is known as the happy hormone.

Then we have another neurotransmitter, gamma-aminobutyric acid (GABA), which is produced in the gut and has the main function of controlling anxiety, stress, and fear. Research indicates that probiotics can decrease fear and anxiety by increasing the production of GABA in the gut (Janik et al., 2016).

## Gut Microbes Produce Other Chemicals That Affect the Brain

The microbes that live in your gut also make other chemicals like short-chain fatty acids (SCFA), and they do this by digesting fiber. Some of these SCFAs are butyrate, propionate, and acetate, and one of their main functions in the brain is to reduce appetite. Consuming propionate was shown to decrease food intake and also decrease brain activity, which is related to the reward it gets from consuming high-energy foods (Byrne et al., 2016).

The other SCFA, butyrate, and the microbes responsible for its production are all involved in the formation of the blood-brain barrier (BBB). This is an important function to shield the brain from toxic substances that may be in the blood, filter compounds from the brain into the blood, and supply brain tissues with the required nutrients.

## Gut Microbes Act on Inflammation

It turns out that gut microbes also play a role in the immune system by controlling what comes in and what goes out of your body, which, in turn, plays a role in inflammation (Robertson, 2023). There's an inflammatory toxin that's made by certain bacteria called lipopolysaccharide (LPS). LPS can cause inflammation if too much of it leaks from the gut to the blood in those diagnosed with a leaky gut. Research shows that high levels of LPS in the blood combined with inflammation could cause brain disorders such as dementia, depression, and schizophrenia (Kelly et al., 2015). This is strong evidence that what goes on in the gut influences what happens in the brain.

**How What You Eat Affects Your Symptoms**

The foods you eat are important throughout your life, but it becomes even more crucial what you choose to include in your diet when you reach menopause for various reasons, including help with managing the menopause symptoms. Dr. Pattimakiel, who is a women's health specialist, recommends a diet rich in protein, vegetables, and calcium at this stage. The Mediterranean diet, which we discussed earlier, caters to that. She also warns against doing anything that's extreme and recommends adopting a lifestyle that's sustainable over the long term (Cleveland Clinic, 2022b).

FOOD TO EAT

**Dairy**

As estrogen levels fall, the risk of osteoporosis and bone fractures increases during menopause. That's why we need dairy because it supplies our bodies with calcium, which is great for bone health. A study conducted by Durosier-Izrat et al. (2017) on 750 women found that women who ate more dairy and animal protein showed significantly higher bone density than those who didn't.

Dairy may also promote deeper sleep in women, as shown in a study of those who ate foods high in glycine, an amino acid present in dairy (Parazzini, 2015).

There's also research that indicates that dairy may decrease the risk of going into early menopause (Purdue-Smithe et al., 2017).

Great sources of calcium are cottage cheese, yogurt, cow's milk, skim milk, and low-fat cheese, and according to Dr. Pattimakiel, we should be aiming for 1200–1500 mg a day to get optimal nutrition (Cleveland Clinic, 2022b).

**Healthy Fats**

Some data indicates that omega-3 fatty acids may decrease menopause symptoms like hot flashes and night sweats (Patade et al., 2008). However, another review of studies proved inconclusive because not all studies showed this effect on hot flashes.

Some of the foods you can include in your diet as sources of omega-3 fatty acids are mackerel, salmon, fatty fish, and anchovies. Flaxseeds, hemp seeds, and chia seeds are also great sources.

## Whole Grains

Research shows that a diet that consists mainly of whole grains reduces the risk of premature death, heart disease, and cancer (Aune et al., 2016). In another study that enrolled 11,000 post-menopausal women, 4.7 grams of whole grains per 2,000 daily calories decreased the risk of premature death by 17% when compared to only 1.3 grams per day (Jacobs et al., 2000).

Excellent sources of whole grains are brown rice, rye, quinoa, barley, and whole wheat bread. Whole grains nourish the body with fiber and B vitamins like niacin, thiamine, pantothenic acid, and riboflavin.

## High-quality Protein

In a study that enrolled menopausal women, those who took 5 grams of collagen had better bone mineral density (BMD) than those who didn't (König et al., 2018). Remember, BMD is one of the things that suffers during menopause due to the decline in estrogen. Collagen is the most abundant protein in our bodies.

The recommended daily allowance (RDA) of protein for women over 50 is 0.45–0.55 grams of protein daily per pound of body weight (Rizzoli et al., 2014). Our total daily calorie intake should include 10–35% protein for optimal health.

Try including these foods in your diets, which are great sources of protein: meat, eggs, fish, dairy, tofu, turkey, and legumes.

## Fruits & Vegetables

The Dietary Guidelines for Americans (USDA, 2020) recommend that half of your plate be filled with fruits and vegetables, as these will nourish your body with fiber, vitamins, minerals, and antioxidants that fight illnesses.

In a large study of over 17,000 menopausal women, those who ate more fruits and vegetables, soy, and fiber reduced their episodes of hot flashes by 19% (Kroenke et al., 2012). Cruciferous vegetables are worth a special mention. Broccoli may be able to increase the type of estrogen that provides protection from breast cancer and decrease the type that is linked to an increased risk of breast cancer, according to research by Fowke et al. (2000).

Another fruit that is worth a special mention is dark berries. There is research that indicates that these fruits may be able to lower blood pressure in menopausal women (Feresin et al., 2017). In this study, only 25 grams of freeze-dried berries were required to show this effect.

Grape seed extract has also been found to help alleviate the symptoms of menopause, such as hot flashes, sleep disturbances, and depression (Terauchi et al., 2014).

## Foods That Contain Phytoestrogen

Phytoestrogen is the compound that acts as estrogen in our bodies, and the foods that contain these compounds are chickpeas, soybeans, peanuts, barley, flaxseeds, grapes, plums, berries, and black and green tea. A review of studies showed that postmenopausal women who took a supplement of soy isoflavone for about four weeks increased their estradiol levels by about 14% compared to those who didn't, though this wasn't a significant difference (Hooper et al., 2009).

There's also research that indicates that phytoestrogens, especially red clover and isoflavone supplements, may lower the incidence of hot flashes (Chen et al., 2014).

## FOODS TO AVOID

Let's start with the two culprits: processed carbs and added sugars. Both of these types of foods raise blood sugar quickly when eaten. High blood sugar, along with insulin resistance and metabolic syndrome, are associated with a high incidence of hot flashes (Cagnacci et al., 2011). Keeping these to a minimum in your diet, or below 10% as recommended by the US guidelines, should help ward off vasomotor symptoms.

### Alcohol and Caffeine

There is research that shows that both alcohol and caffeine increase the severity of hot flashes, though they don't increase their frequency (Kandiah & Amend, 2010). A different study suggested that caffeine may lower the incidence, so it's best that you judge for yourself, as each individual may get a different result. I would advise that you exercise moderation when it comes to these two.

**Spicy Food**

Spicy foods may increase the incidence of hot flashes (Hunter et al., 2012) and increase anxiety (Stefanopoulou et al., 2013), although the latter was associated with pre-existing poor health. Again, it's best that you judge for yourself on this one and see if this happens to you after eating spicy food.

**Salty Food**

A high salt intake is associated with a lower BMD in post-menopausal women, with just 2 mg of salt per day increasing the risk of low BMD by 28% (Kwon et al., 2017). Also, controlling your salt intake may improve your mood (Torres & Nowson, 2012).

## MOOD-BOOSTING FOODS

The following foods may help improve your mood:

**Fatty Fish**

Two types of omega-3s have been shown through research to decrease levels of depression: docosahexaenoic acid (DHA) and eicosapentaenoic acid (EPA). Fatty fish such as salmon and albacore tuna are excellent sources of these omega-3s. Getting your omega-3s from fish oil may also help decrease depression (Yang et al., 2018).

Lastly, omega-3s may also play a key role in brain development (Bozzatello et al., 2016).

## Dark Chocolate

Dark chocolate may boost your mood because it contains other feel-good compounds like caffeine, N-acylethanolamine, which is a compound similar to cannabinoids, and theobromine. It's also loaded with health-promoting flavonoids that may increase the flow of blood to your brain, improve brain health, and reduce inflammation, all contributing to mood regulation (Scholey & Owen, 2013).

Let's not forget that chocolate is a pleasure to taste and smell. Try to stick to dark chocolate instead of milk chocolate, as the latter is higher in sugar and fat, and try to limit yourself to two squares at a time since chocolate is high in calories.

## Fermented Foods

Here, we are talking about foods like kimchi, kombucha, kefir, yogurt, and sauerkraut, which supply your body with probiotics created during fermentation. The live microorganisms promote the growth of healthy bacteria in your gut, which then increases your serotonin levels (Yano et al., 2015), thus boosting your mood. Research also shows that healthy gut bacteria are associated with lower depression rates (O'Mahony et al., 2015).

## Bananas

Bananas provide your body with sugar and fiber, but this is not bad sugar. When sugar is paired with fiber like this, it is slowly released into your bloodstream, giving you stable sugar levels throughout the day and better control over your mood. Also, the B-6 vitamin found in bananas plays an important role in synthesizing dopamine and serotonin, your feel-good hormones. Green bananas are also great sources of prebiotics that feed your gut's healthy bacteria and ultimately improve your brain function (Huang et al., 2019).

## Oats

Oats are an excellent source of fiber, and like bananas, the slow release of sugar in your body is aided by fiber. Research shows that those who eat 1.5–6 grams of fiber in the morning report better mood and energy for the day (Evans Kreider et al., 2017). Oats are also a great source of iron, and those with iron deficiencies may experience mood swings, sluggishness, and fatigue, which iron helps alleviate.

## Berries

Berries are a great source of antioxidants and phenolic compounds, both of which combat oxidative stress, which often results from an imbalance of harmful compounds in our bodies (Olas, 2018). Oxidative stress contributes to our bodies' rapid aging.

Anthocyanins, a pigment found in berries, could lower the risk of depression by 39% (Godos et al., 2018).

## CONCLUSION

In this chapter, I discussed the impact of lifestyle on your general well-being, specifically exercise, sleep, and diet. The main reason behind this was to show how making small tweaks to each of those areas can alleviate some of your menopause symptoms. I also revisited the relationship between the food you eat and your mental health, the mind-gut relationship, and suggested some of the foods that you can safely add to your diet to reap the most health benefits, as well as those that you should avoid.

These are all outward changes that you can easily incorporate into your lifestyle. The next chapter, however, takes you on an inward journey to see what changes can be made there to help you not only embrace but navigate this phase of life.

# 7

# A JOURNEY INWARD

*Nothing in the world is permanent, we are foolish when we ask anything to last, but surely we are more foolish not to take delight when it lasts.*

— SOMERSET MAUGHAM

## MENOPAUSE AND THE IDEA OF TRANSIENT LIFE

All living things move through phases—birth, growth, decline, and renewal. Our bodies change, just like the seasons change, and this marks the different chapters in our life journey. Menopause is just one of those chapters or phases of life that offers you real physical evidence that nothing is permanent. Throughout this book, we have been emphasizing the need to shift our perspective from seeing this phase as a crisis to embracing it as a positive experience. This is the *Radiant Shift Method.*

Rather than resisting or fearing menopause, acknowledging it as a natural progression can bring peace and acceptance. This acceptance often brings a deeper appreciation for every moment and stage of life. While youth and fertility are often celebrated, they are temporary states, just like every other phase of life.

The Buddhists have what is called the *first dharma seal of the law of impermanence* to remind us that everything we see is impermanent. They also use the term *anicca*, which means "impermanence," to denote the idea of continuous change that we human beings go through. In their view, when we expect certain aspects of our lives, like our career, beauty, wealth, family, and so on, to be fixed or permanent, we intensify the pain of loss and disappointment that we will feel when said things change. Confino and Hữu (2021) remind us that according to the law of impermanence, "whatever we are feeling today will change tomorrow".

## HOW CAN EMBRACING THE IDEA OF IMPERMANENCE HELP US?

According to Buddhism, accepting the impermanence of things can liberate us, as it opens us up to endless possibilities (Nash, 2016). For them, the whole purpose of life is to free yourself from the cyclic process of suffering that you bring upon yourself when you cling to temporary things by achieving a state of enlightenment, or nirvana (Nash, 2016).

Brady (2020) names one benefit of embracing impermanence as allowing us to gain peace, equanimity, and confidence. He advises that the sooner we embrace it, the less we will suffer in the future when it's thrust upon us. According to Chakravorty (2020), accepting life's impermanence allows us to grow, adapt, survive, and thrive. He further asserts that this allows us to reflect, respond, and add value not only to ourselves but to those around us.

Thich Nhat Hanh wrote (2015):

> *If you suffer, it is not because things are impermanent. It is because you believe things are permanent. When a flower dies, you don't suffer much because you understand that flowers are impermanent... If you look deeply into impermanence, you will do your best to make her happy right now. Aware of impermanence, you become positive, loving, and wise. Impermanence is good news. Without impermanence, nothing would be possible. With impermanence, every door is open for change. Impermanence is an instrument for our liberation.*

What we know for sure is that only death is permanent. Menopause offers a poignant reminder that you are still very much alive. And that is a gift.

## A TIME FOR REINVENTION: YOUR UNIQUE PATH POSTMENOPAUSE

For many women, life before menopause may have followed a script—perhaps one that society, family, or tradition laid out. There were expectations to meet, milestones to achieve by certain ages, roles to fill, and paths to follow. Now is the perfect time to ask yourself, "Whose life have you been living?" "What are your passions, dreams, and desires that have been waiting patiently in the wings?" The point isn't to dwell on the past but rather to eagerly and genuinely embrace the future. This reinvention is not necessarily about becoming someone new, but rather about returning to who you truly are at your core. When you shed the layers of external expectations, you can become who you really are meant to be.

## So What Does Reinventing Yourself Look Like?

First things first, reinventing yourself doesn't mean starting anew, but rather starting from a new point in your life, this time with different goals, dreams, and values than when you were younger.

(Clendenin, 2023) suggests 11 ways you can reinvent yourself at 50, and I will summarize them here:

- Learn new skills. Things are moving at the speed of light; every day there's new technology to master, and we have to keep up. Find websites that offer free courses and develop your skills.
- Live an authentic life. Don't be like those people whose biggest regret on their dying bed is that they lived to make other people happy and not themselves. Use reinvention to help you transform from surviving to living your best life.

- Heal your wounds. Work on healing past hurts and traumas. This could involve going to psychotherapy or joining a yoga or meditation class.
- Be intentional with your time and energy. Pick a charity cause that you really care about. For a long time, you participated in things because you had to, not because you deeply cared for them.
- Seek mentors and inspiration. Find those who have done what you're trying to do, and ask them to mentor you as you chart your way forward. Also, consider being a mentor to others using the skills you have acquired.
- Craft a long-term plan. Set long-term goals. What do you want to achieve in five, 10, or 15 years from now?
- Get support from loved ones. You increase your chances of succeeding when you have the support of those closest to you.
- Let go of what doesn't serve you. This helps you reach new heights. It includes things like letting go of bad habits and self-doubt.
- Try different things. Who said you couldn't get on the next TikTok challenge? Or try out your recipe for cookies and sell them at the next menopause support group or church.
- Focus on what you want. Focus on who you want to be and on building those aspects of yourself that help you be that person. You control the timeline, so use it to your advantage.
- Learn to fail forward. Take every *failure* as a lesson instead of beating yourself up about it. When you fall, learn to get

up and keep moving forward by using the lessons to better yourself. Remember when Col. Sanders discovered his secret chicken recipe at 65? So what's stopping you?

## CONCLUSION

The last point I want to make before closing this chapter is that it's never too late to reinvent yourself, and there are many examples of women who have done this in our time. One of those is Margaret Skoglund, who, when COVID-19 shutdowns made it impossible to perform live Broadway shows, came up with the idea of putting together and selling virtual shows to companies for corporate events as a way to alleviate stress and entertain employees during the pandemic. If you want to reinvent yourself, I would recommend putting together a vision board, and you can do this with the help of Pinterest too. Find examples of all the things that speak to you, and create a vision board that sparks a beautiful idea of what you want to do going forward and how you want to live your best life.

# 8

# BEING A PILLAR: SUPPORTING THE MENOPAUSAL WOMEN IN YOUR LIFE

*I find the best way to love someone is not to change them, but instead, help them reveal the greatest version of themselves.*

— STEVE MARABOLI

Menopause brings about a myriad of physical, emotional, and mental changes. By providing support and understanding during menopause, you're empowering the woman in your life to face challenges head-on and embrace the next phase of her life with confidence.

## WHAT TO EXPECT

The first thing you need to do is educate yourself about what your partner is going through so that you may be best able to help them navigate these tumultuous waters. Expect mood swings, hot flashes, night sweats, depression, anxiety, and other physical changes.

## WHEN TO EXPECT IT?

The average age of menopause is 51 in the US, but menopause can start as early as seven years before they receive their last menses and can last up to five years after their last period (Cleveland Clinic, 2021c).

## WHAT CAUSES THEM?

These are caused by the fluctuating levels of the hormones estrogen and progesterone, which affect the ability of a woman's body to regulate her temperature and other processes. The most common symptoms mentioned above are hot flashes, night sweats, mood swings, brain fog, and depression. Other women may also experience vaginal dryness, bleeding, and pain when having sex.

## EVERY WOMAN EXPERIENCES MENOPAUSE DIFFERENTLY

Please know that although most women go through the well-known symptoms of menopause—hot flashes, night sweats, mood swings, and depression—not all women are the same, and some may not go through that much. Remember that women's menstrual cycles are different, and so will their experience of menopause.

## IT'S NOT ALWAYS BETTER THAN A PERIOD

As a man, do not automatically assume that just because a woman has stopped menstruating, she is happy about it, because it isn't necessarily better than getting your period. One woman was quoted saying, "It felt like dementia and puberty had a kid together!" (Brusie, 2019).

## THERE WILL BE PHYSICAL CHANGES THAT CAN BE HARD TO HANDLE

Some women genuinely feel that the cons of entering menopause far outweigh the pros of no longer having periods, as they have to deal with lots of new physical changes, including weight gain, abdominal fat, and hair changes, among many other things, during this time.

## THE PMS DOESN'T ALWAYS GO AWAY

Some women report that PMS doesn't always go away with their periods but that instead, life could feel like one long pre-period week—PMS with no end.

## THERE WILL BE SHIFTING

Even the skinniest of women may notice their weight distribution shifting at this time, with most people noticing a pudge around the waist. Gravity also plays a part in how things start shaping up, and you are advised to be sensitive about this subject.

## HOW TO SURVIVE HER MENOPAUSE AND HELP HER TRANSITION THROUGH IT

Dr. Pepper Schwartz (2010) advises men to be sensitive to what their partner is going through instead of being dismissive and saying things like, "It can't be that bad." Instead, see how you can help by maybe bringing her a pitcher of ice-cold water when she's going through a hot flash or doing something similar to that, and don't be disappointed if she rebuffs your offer to help.

**Learn More About Menopause**

I already mentioned above the importance of arming yourself with knowledge, learning as much as possible about why menopause happens, the symptoms, and what treatment options are available out there, including some ways to ease the symptoms at home. This will help you provide the best support for your loved one.

**Prepare for Mood Swings**

Preparing for mood swings means you will be best able to deal with them when they surface. This entails being less judgmental and not taking things personally. How about suggesting a fun activity you can do together to boost her mood?

**Don't Take It Personally**

The sooner you understand that none of this is directed at you, the better. Your partner's distress based on what is happening to her body has nothing to do with you. She may even have some words directed at you, but understand that this isn't her talking and that your relationship isn't falling apart just because she's behaving that way.

### Keep a Sense of Humor but Don't Make Fun of Them

A sense of humor will help lighten the mood and remind your partner that the relationship is still fun, but make sure you're not making jokes about her. Laugh with her, not at her, and whatever you do, don't make jokes about her changing body.

### Be Empathetic

Stand in her shoes for a moment and imagine how you would feel if your body was changing and you were feeling like you were losing the sense of who you are. This will make you more empathetic.

### Talk About It

Opens the lines of communication about what she's going through. Ask her how you may help ease her stress. Suggest healthy and fun activities that you can do together. Similarly, share your feelings if you were hurt by her behavior earlier in a sensitive way.

**Offer to Help**

Being proactive works better than being reactive, which means anticipating situations that add stress to her life and seeing how you can help. If you can see that she's feeling a bit overwhelmed by responsibilities, offer to wash the dishes or cook one night.

**Seek Help if You Need It**

It's always a good idea to talk to a professional if you are not coping with what's going on in your relationship. They may offer some tips and tools to help you manage the stress that you're under. They may also know of a support group that you can join to learn from and gain support from others who are in a similar position.

**Support Her New Goals**

If she wants to start a new hobby, show her support. Is there anything that you can do? If she wants to join a gym, you could join her and get healthy together. Research shows that couples who exercise together are more likely to be consistent and that this improves the relationship (Sackett-Fox et al., 2021).

**Be There for Them**

Be an ever-present pillar of support. This means that when she wants to talk about her feelings, be willing to listen, and when she needs to go to the doctor, offer to go with her.

## Know That Menopause Is Not Forever

Remind yourself that this too shall pass. Take comfort in the fact that this will get better over time.

While the above advice applies to everyone close to the woman who's going through menopause, the next few tips are specifically directed to their partners.

## Keep up the Romance

Just because the woman in your life is going through a season of symptoms that may leave her feeling crabby and uninterested doesn't mean romance is off the table completely. There are many ways to keep the love alive and make her feel beautiful and desirable, such as holding her hand, buying her flowers, etc.

## Be Patient in the Bedroom

Your sex life is one area that is hit the hardest by menopause. This is because low testosterone levels impact her libido, and fluctuating estrogen levels may cause her vagina to feel dry, resulting in painful sex. So she may lose interest in the whole thing. Learn to exercise patience, and if she turns you down, be understanding, as disappointing as that may be. You can try again when she's in a better mood.

**Make Her Feel Beautiful**

A woman who's going through body changes, gaining weight in all the wrong areas, and having gravity take its toll doesn't feel confident. Do your best to remind her that she is beautiful and that you still find her attractive—hold her hand, take her out on a date, caress her hand when you're sitting on the couch—the list is endless.

**"Duck and Cover" Is Not a Relationship Strategy**

Angelo (2017) shares this tip about knowing yourself and playing to your strengths. This means if you are a "Mr. Fix-it," you should find out what you can do to fix things to make her life a bit easier. Maybe she needs ceiling fans installed in every room, or so on. Whatever you do, do not assume you can just take cover for the next few years while she's going through it. Show up and offer support as best as you can.

CONCLUSION

I want to end this chapter by letting you know that I understand the challenges you may be facing right now if you have a loved one who is going through menopause. Take comfort in knowing that millions of others are going through the same thing and that it will pass. Menopause is not forever. In this chapter, we shared some tips to help you navigate this phase of life as best as you can, but the running theme throughout was to *be supportive*. How do you do that? By learning as much as you can about menopause and showing up as best as you can for your loved one who's going through it.

# CONCLUSION

I can't believe that we have come to the end of our book! In conclusion, I want to leave you with this thought: ***Just as the most beautiful and deep colors of the sky aren't revealed at noon, but during sunrise and sunset, a woman's depth, wisdom, and beauty are not confined to her youth.***

Menopause isn't the fading of a woman's light; it's the deepening of her glow.

I wrote this book as a way to invite women all over the world to join me in seeing menopause in a different light. To embrace it as a positive experience rather than something to be dreaded or viewed as a crisis. The message of this book has been built on what I call the Radiant Shift Method, which advocates for a whole-body approach, considering mental, emotional, and physical aspects when addressing symptoms. It emphasizes being kind to yourself, owning your story, and gliding through this stage of life as the radiant human being that you are.

In just eight chapters, we have covered every aspect of what menopause brings into a woman's life, from what symptoms to expect and what causes them to options for treatment. We also shared tips on different ways we can tweak our lifestyle to set us up for the best outcome and prevent lifestyle diseases. We delved into the world of emotions, sex, sensuality, nutrition, and exercise. We also discussed the concept of impermanence, a Buddhist way of living in the present and understanding that all things change, and with that, we discussed various ways to reinvent yourself.

The last chapter was a bonus chapter for the people close to us, family and friends, to arm them with knowledge and strategies of how they can best provide support to us while we are going through the great metamorphosis. I call it metamorphosis simply because it's a period of transition, as a butterfly emerges out of its cocoon to become the most beautiful version of itself.

Remember, every phase of life brings its own kind of power. Menopause is not the end; it's a radiant new beginning. Own your glow. Own your journey.

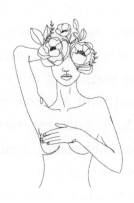

# NAVIGATING TOGETHER

Now that you've gathered all the tools to go through menopause, it's time to share your newfound wisdom and guide other women to discover the same helpful insights.

By sharing your honest thoughts about this book on Amazon, you're not just leaving a review; you'll show other women where they can find the information they're looking for.

Your assistance is truly appreciated. The journey through menopause becomes more manageable when we share what we've learned.

Scan the QR code below to leave your review on Amazon:

Thank you for your help.

Warm regards,
Kate Hartwell

# REFERENCES

Abramson, A. (2022, November 1). *Meditation techniques to help with menopause symptoms.* Stripes. https://iamstripes.com/blogs/mental-health/medita tion-techniques-to-help-with-menopause-symptoms

Ageless Restoration. (n.d.). *The history of menopause.* Ageless Restoration. https://www.balancehormoneoklahoma.com/blog/the-history-of-menopause

Agencies. (2016, March 8). *Sedentary lifestyle might worsen menopausal symptoms.* TheHealthSite.com. https://www.thehealthsite.com/news/seden tary-lifestyle-might-worsen-menopausal-symptoms-364185/

Albarda, V. (2021, October 13). *50 Journal Prompts for a midlife woman's journey to self-discovery.* Midlife-A-Go-Go. https://www.midlifeagogo.com/50-journal-prompts-midlife-womans-journey-self-discovery/

Aletheia. (2021, August 3). *How to be sensual (and increase your sexual confidence).* LonerWolf. https://lonerwolf.com/how-to-sensuality/

American Academy of Dermatology Association. (n.d.). *Caring for your skin in menopause.* American Academy of Dermatology Association. https://www. aad.org/public/everyday-care/skin-care-secrets/anti-aging/skin-care-during-menopause

Anderson, K. (2021, September 22). *I'm a middle-aged woman. Here's what the media still gets wrong about us.* HuffPost. https://www.huffpost.com/entry/middle-aged-women-myths-tv-shows_n_6148c9bbe4b0efa77f8386c4

Angelo, J. (2017, June 16). *Menopause help for husbands: 6 tips on how to help your midlife wife.* Gennev. https://www.gennev.com/education/menopause-help-for-husbands

Aune, D., Keum, N., Giovannucci, E., Fadnes, L. T., Boffetta, P., Greenwood, D. C., Tonstad, S., Vatten, L. J., Riboli, E., & Norat, T. (2016, June 14). Whole grain consumption and risk of cardiovascular disease, cancer, and all-cause and cause-specific mortality: systematic review and dose-response meta-analysis of prospective studies. *BMJ*, i2716. https://doi.org/10.1136/bmj.i2716

Australian Institute of Health & Welfare. (2016). *How lifestyle choices affect our health.* Australian Institute of Health & Welfare. https://www.aihw.gov.au/

getmedia/0ea3cb23-34c3-4e3b-8a20-8c1c0cde6586/ah16-factsheet-lifestylechoices.pdf.aspx

Australian Menopause Society. (2019). *Lifestyle and behavioral modifications for menopausal symptoms.* Australian Menopause Society. https://www.menopause.org.au/hp/information-sheets/lifestyle-and-behavioural-modifications-for-menopausal-symptoms

Avis, N. E., Coeytaux, R. R., Isom, S., Prevette, K., & Morgan, T. (2016). Acupuncture in Menopause (AIM) study. *Menopause, 23*(6), 626–637. https://doi.org/10.1097/gme.0000000000000597

Axe, J. (2023, April 27). *Best menopause supplements & diet to relieve symptoms.* Dr. Axe. https://draxe.com/health/menopause-supplements-diet/

Baron, J. (2022, November 29). *The relationship between menopause and stress.* Katie Couric Media. https://katiecouric.com/health/wellness/the-relationship-between-menopause-and-stress/

Belcher, N. (November 2, 2023). *Cortisol levels: How it impacts menopause symptoms.* Winona. https://bywinona.com/journal/cortisol-levels-how-they-impact-weight-anxiety-and-stress-in-menopause

Bennett, J. (2014, August 7). *Stop telling women their most valuable asset is their youth.* Time. https://time.com/3087527/stop-telling-women-our-most-valuable-asset-is-our-youth/

Better Health Channel. (2022, November 21). *Menopause and weight gain.* Better Health Channel. https://www.betterhealth.vic.gov.au/health/conditionsandtreatments/menopause-and-weight-gain

Bonanno, L., Metro, D., Papa, M., Finzi, G., Maviglia, A., Sottile, F., Corallo, F., & Manasseri, L. (2019). Assessment of sleep and obesity in adults and children. *Medicine, 98*(46), e17642. https://doi.org/10.1097/md.0000000000017642

Boomkens, D. (2020, May 22). *Famous women on aging.* AndBloom. https://www.andbloom.amsterdam/famous-women-on-aging/

Born, L., Koren, G., Lin, E., & Steiner, M. (2008). A new, female-specific irritability rating scale. *Journal of Psychiatry & Neuroscience: JPN, 33*(4), 344–354. https://www.ncbi.nlm.nih.gov/pmc/articles/PMC2440789/

Bozzatello, P., Brignolo, E., De Grandi, E., & Bellino, S. (2016). Supplementation with omega-3 fatty acids in psychiatric disorders: A Review of Literature Data. *Journal of Clinical Medicine, 5*(8), 67. https://doi.org/10.3390/jcm5080067

Bracy, K. (2023, April 5). *A guide on how to support partners during menopause.*

Verywell Health. https://www.verywellhealth.com/supporting-your-part ner-during-menopause-2322673#citation-7

Brady, A. (2020, November 19). *Impermanence—life's great wake-up call.* Chopra. https://chopra.com/articles/impermanence-lifes-great-wake-up-call

Bravo, J. A., Forsythe, P., Chew, M. V., Escaravage, E., Savignac, H. M., Dinan, T. G., Bienenstock, J., & Cryan, J. F. (2011). Ingestion of Lactobacillus strain regulates emotional behavior and central GABA receptor expression in a mouse via the vagus nerve. *Proceedings of the National Academy of Sciences, 108*(38), 16050–16055. https://doi.org/10.1073/pnas.1102999108

British Menopause Society. (2022). *Testosterone replacement in menopause.* British Menopause Society. https://thebms.org.uk/wp-content/uploads/2022/12/08-BMS-TfC-Testosterone-replacement-in-menopause-DEC2022-A.pdf

Brown, B. (2018, May 24). *The midlife unraveling.* Brené Brown. https://brene brown.com/articles/2018/05/24/the-midlife-unraveling

Brusie, C. (August 12, 2019). *8 things women want men to know about menopause.* Healthline. https://www.healthline.com/health/8-things-every-woman-wants-men-to-know-about-menopause

Byrne, C. S., Chambers, E. S., Alhabeeb, H., Chhina, N., Morrison, D. J., Preston, T., Tedford, C., Fitzpatrick, J., Irani, C., Busza, A., Garcia-Perez, I., Fountana, S., Holmes, E., Goldstone, A. P., & Frost, G. S. (2016). Increased colonic propionate reduces anticipatory reward responses in the human striatum to high-energy foods. *The American Journal of Clinical Nutrition, 104*(1), 5–14. https://doi.org/10.3945/ajcn.115.126706

Cagnacci, A., Cannoletta, M., Palma, F., Zanin, R., Xholli, A., & Volpe, A. (2011). Menopausal symptoms and risk factors for cardiovascular disease in postmenopause. *Climacteric, 15*(2), 157–162. https://doi.org/10.3109/13697137.2011.617852

Calra, R. (2022, October 18). *Menopause, not an end to youth but beginning of a new phase!!* The Statesman. https://www.thestatesman.com/lifestyle/menopause-not-an-end-to-youth-but-beginning-of-a-new-phase-1503122827.html

Carnegy, A. (2016, December). *Fertility and femininity.* Medical Travel. https://www.medicaltravelczech.com/blog/ivf-egg-donation/fertility-and-femininity

Cedars Sinai. (n.d.). *Stroke.* Cedars Sinai. https://www.cedars-sinai.org/health-library/diseases-and-conditions/s/stroke-1.html

Chakravorty, D. (2020, November 25). *The gifts of impermanence.* Medium. https://rahul-debanjan.medium.com/the-gifts-of-impermanence-aa43d7ea7852

Chen, M-n., Lin, C-c., & Liu, C-f. (2014). Efficacy of phytoestrogens for menopausal symptoms: a meta-analysis and systematic review. *Climacteric, 18*(2), 260–269. https://doi.org/10.3109/13697137.2014.966241

Clendenin, R. (2023, March 8). *Second act at 50: How to make the most of your midlife reinvention.* Retirely. https://retirely.co/reinvent-yourself-50

Cleveland Clinic. (2021a, May 10). *Postmenopause.* Cleveland Clinic. https://my.clevelandclinic.org/health/diseases/21837-postmenopause

Cleveland Clinic. (2021b, June 28). *Hormone therapy for menopause symptoms.* Cleveland Clinic. https://my.clevelandclinic.org/health/treatments/15245-hormone-therapy-for-menopause-symptoms

Cleveland Clinic. (2021c, October 5). *Menopause.* Cleveland Clinic. https://my.clevelandclinic.org/health/diseases/21841-menopause

Cleveland Clinic. (2022a, January 11). *Vagus Nerve.* Cleveland Clinic. https://my.clevelandclinic.org/health/body/22279-vagus-nerve

Cleveland Clinic. (2022b, July 5). *Menopause diet: What to eat to help manage symptoms.* Cleveland Clinic. https://health.clevelandclinic.org/menopause-diet/

Cleveland Clinic. (2022c, December 29). *Progesterone.* Cleveland Clinic. https://my.clevelandclinic.org/health/body/24562-progesterone#:

Codrington, K. (2021, May 26). *Three breathing techniques to help with menopause symptoms.* Kate Codrington. https://www.katecodrington.co.uk/three-breathing-techniques-to-help-with-menopause-symptoms/

Confino, J., & Hữu, C. (Hosts). (2021–present). Lessons in impermanence: how to handle life when everything changes [Audio podcast episode]. In *The Way Out Is In.* Plum Village. https://plumvillage.org/podcast/lessons-in-impermanence-how-to-handle-life-when-everything-changes

Dalal, P., & Agarwal, M. (2015). Postmenopausal syndrome. *Indian Journal of Psychiatry, 57*(6), 222. https://doi.org/10.4103/0019-5545.161483

Davidson, K. (2020, February 5). *9 Healthy Foods That Lift Your Mood.* Healthline. https://www.healthline.com/nutrition/mood-food

Drake, C. L., Kalmbach, D. A., Arnedt, J. T., Cheng, P., Tonnu, C. V., Cuamatzi-Castelan, A., & Fellman-Couture, C. (2018). Treating chronic insomnia in postmenopausal women: a randomized clinical trial comparing cognitive-behavioral therapy for insomnia, sleep restriction therapy, and sleep hygiene education. *Sleep, 42*(2). https://doi.org/10.1093/sleep/zsy217

Durosier-Izart, C., Biver, E., Merminod, F., van Rietbergen, B., Chevalley, T., Herrmann, F. R., Ferrari, S. L., & Rizzoli, R. (2017). Peripheral skeleton bone strength is positively correlated with total and dairy protein intakes in healthy postmenopausal women. *The American Journal of Clinical Nutrition, 105*(2), 513–525. https://doi.org/10.3945/ajcn.116.134676

Durward, E. (2019, November 11). *5 menopause symptoms made worse by stress.* A.Vogel. https://www.avogel.co.uk/health/menopause/videos/5-menopause-symptoms-made-worse-by-stress/

Earnest, C. P., Johannsen, N. M., Swift, D. L., Lavie, C. J., Blair, S. N., & Church, T. S. (2013). Dose effect of cardiorespiratory exercise on metabolic syndrome in postmenopausal women. *The American Journal of Cardiology, 111*(12), 1805–1811. https://doi.org/10.1016/j.amjcard.2013.02.037

El Khoudary, S. R., Greendale, G., Crawford, S. L., Avis, N. E., Brooks, M. M., Thurston, R. C., Karvonen-Gutierrez, C., Waetjen, L. E., & Matthews, K. (2019). The menopause transition and women's health at midlife. *Menopause, 26*(10), 1213–1227. https://doi.org/10.1097/gme.0000000000001424

Elite Daily. (2014, June 2). *The timeless qualities women have that men will always find attractive.* The Good Men Project. https://goodmenproject.com/featured-content/the-timeless-qualities-women-have-that-men-will-always-find-attractive-grgs/

Endocrine Society. (2022, January 24). *Menopause.* Endocrine Society. https://www.endocrine.org/patient-engagement/endocrine-library/menopause

Evans Kreider, K., Pereira, K., & Padilla, B. I. (2017). Practical approaches to diagnosing, treating and preventing hypoglycemia in diabetes. *Diabetes Therapy, 8*(6), 1427–1435. https://doi.org/10.1007/s13300-017-0325-9

Farzaneh, F., Fatehi, S., Sohrabi, M.-R., & Alizadeh, K. (2013). The effect of oral evening primrose oil on menopausal hot flashes: a randomized clinical trial. *Archives of Gynecology and Obstetrics, 288*(5), 1075–1079. https://doi.org/10.1007/s00404-013-2852-6

Feresin, R. G., Johnson, S. A., Pourafshar, S., Campbell, J. C., Jaime, S. J., Navaei, N., Elam, M. L., Akhavan, N. S., Alvarez-Alvarado, S., Tenenbaum,

G., Brummel-Smith, K., Salazar, G., Figueroa, A., & Arjmandi, B. H. (2017). Impact of daily strawberry consumption on blood pressure and arterial stiffness in pre- and stage 1-hypertensive postmenopausal women: a randomized controlled trial. *Food & Function, 8*(11), 4139–4149. https://doi.org/10.1039/c7fo01183k

Forth. (2020, October 28). *Menopause hormones - what are they and how do they change?* Forth. https://www.forthwithlife.co.uk/blog/menopause-hormones/

Fowke, J. H., Longcope, C., & Hebert, J. R. (2000). Brassica vegetable consumption shifts estrogen metabolism in healthy postmenopausal women. *Cancer Epidemiology, Biomarkers & Prevention: A Publication of the American Association for Cancer Research, Cosponsored by the American Society of Preventive Oncology, 9*(8), 773–779. https://pubmed.ncbi.nlm.nih.gov/10952093/

Freeman, E. W. (2015). Depression in the menopause transition: risks in the changing hormone milieu as observed in the general population. *Women's Midlife Health, 1*(1). https://doi.org/10.1186/s40695-015-0002-y

Gaskell, A. (2023, January 10). *Unfair stereotypes of middle-aged women hold them back at work.* Forbes. https://www.forbes.com/sites/adigaskell/2023/01/10/unfair-stereotypes-of-middle-aged-women-hold-them-back-at-work/?sh=5ffe47973adc

Godos, J., Castellano, S., Ray, S., Grosso, G., & Galvano, F. (2018). Dietary polyphenol intake and depression: results from the Mediterranean Healthy Eating, Lifestyle and Aging (MEAL) Study. *Molecules, 23*(5), 999. https://doi.org/10.3390/molecules23050999

Gomstyn, A. (2019). *Food for your mood: How what you eat affects your mental health.* Aetna. https://www.aetna.com/health-guide/food-affects-mental-health.html

Gorrepati, P. (2019, May 1). What's hormones got to do with it? The medicalization of menopause in postwar America. *Hektoen International - a Journal of Medical Humanities.* https://hekint.org/2019/05/01/whats-hormones-got-to-do-with-it-the-medicalization-of-menopause-in-postwar-america/

Goss, A. M., Chandler-Laney, P. C., Ovalle, F., Goree, L. L., Azziz, R., Desmond, R. A., Wright Bates, G., & Gower, B. A. (2014). Effects of a eucaloric reduced-carbohydrate diet on body composition and fat distribution in women with PCOS. *Metabolism, 63*(10), 1257–1264. https://doi. org/10.1016/j.metabol.2014.07.007

Grantham, J. P., & Henneberg, M. (2014). The estrogen hypothesis of obesity. *PLoS ONE, 9*(6). https://doi.org/10.1371/journal.pone.0099776

Groves, M. (2018, November 23). *Menopause diet: how what you eat affects your symptoms.* Healthline. https://www.healthline.com/nutrition/menopause-diet#menopause

Gunter, J. (2021, May 15). Menopause is not the end of a journey – it's crossing a bridge to something new. *The Globe and Mail.* https://www. theglobeandmail.com/opinion/article-menopause-is-not-the-end-of-a-journey-its-crossing-a-bridge-to/

Hames, M. V. (2023, May 5). *Mayo Clinic minute: Why alcohol and menopause can be a dangerous mix.* Mayo Clinic News Network. https://newsnetwork. mayoclinic.org/discussion/mayo-clinic-minute-why-alcohol-and-menopause-can-be-a-dangerous-mix/

Hampton, D. (2022, March 22). *Your mindset shapes your life - for better or worse.* The Best Brain Possible. https://thebestbrainpossible.com/mindset-growth-fixed-success-mental-health/

Hartescu, I., Morgan, K., & Stevinson, C. D. (2015). Increased physical activity improves sleep and mood outcomes in inactive people with insomnia: a randomized controlled trial. *Journal of Sleep Research, 24*(5), 526–534. https://doi.org/10.1111/jsr.12297

HCA Healthcare UK. (2023). *18 signs of the menopause you might have missed.* HCA Healthcare UK. https://www.hcahealthcare.co.uk/blogs/18-signs-of-the-menopause-you-might-have-missed

Hepburn, A. (n.d.). *Audrey Hepburn quotes.* Goodreads. https://www. goodreads.com/quotes/133783-and-the-beauty-of-a-woman-with-pass ing-years-only

Herrera, K. (2019, December 4). *Hormones and emotional health.* Women's International Pharmacy. https://www.womensinternational.com/blog/ hormones-and-emotional-health/

Hodis, H. N., & Mack, W. J. (2022). Menopausal hormone replacement therapy and reduction of all-cause mortality and cardiovascular disease. *The Cancer Journal, 28*(3), 208–223. https://doi.org/10.1097/ppo.0000000000000591

Hoffman, M. (2022, November 28). *Estrogen and women's emotions.* WebMD. https://www.webmd.com/women/estrogen-and-womens-emotions

Hooper, L., Ryder, J. J., Kurzer, M. S., Lampe, J. W., Messina, M. J., Phipps, W. R., & Cassidy, A. (2009). Effects of soy protein and isoflavones on circulating hormone concentrations in pre- and post-menopausal women: a systematic review and meta-analysis. *Human Reproduction Update, 15*(4), 423–440. https://doi.org/10.1093/humupd/dmp010

Hormone and Wellness Center of Texas. (n.d.). *10 myths about hormone replacement therapy.* Hormone Wellness Center. https://hwcoftexas.com/10-hormone-replacement-myths/

Hormone Health. (n.d.). *The most common myths about HRT – busted!* Hormone Health. https://hormonehealth.co.uk/the-most-common-myths-about-hrt-busted

Hornung, S. (2019). Crafting task and cognitive job boundaries to enhance self-determination, impact, meaning, and competence at work. *Behavioral Sciences, 9*(12), 136. https://doi.org/10.3390/bs9120136

Huang, T.-T., Lai, J.-B., Du, Y.-L., Xu, Y., Ruan, L.-M., & Hu, S.-H. (2019). Current understanding of gut microbiota in mood disorders: an update of human studies. *Frontiers in Genetics, 10.* https://doi.org/10.3389/fgene.2019.00098

Huizen, J. (2023, August 1). *Everything you should know about menopause.* Healthline. https://www.healthline.com/health/menopause#causes

Hulem, R. (2013, March 5). *Does menopause cause midlife crisis?* Poise. https://www.poise.com/en-us/advice-and-support/menopause/midlife-crisis

Hunt, A. (2021, September 1). *Menopause support groups—how to find the right community for you.* Woman & Home. https://www.womanandhome.com/health-and-wellbeing/menopause-help-support-forums-327512/

Hunter, M. S., Gupta, P., Chedraui, P., Blümel, J. E., Tserotas, K., Aguirre, W., Palacios, S., & Sturdee, D. W. (2012). The International Menopause Study of Climate, Altitude, Temperature (IMS-CAT) and vasomotor symptoms. *Climacteric, 16*(1), 8–16. https://doi.org/10.3109/13697137.2012.699563

Infantino, M. (2008). The prevalence and pattern of gastroesophageal reflux symptoms in perimenopausal and menopausal women. *Journal of the American Academy of Nurse Practitioners, 20*(5), 266–272. https://doi.org/10.1111/j.1745-7599.2008.00316.x

Jackson, S. E., Kirschbaum, C., & Steptoe, A. (2017). Hair cortisol and adiposity in a population-based sample of 2,527 men and women aged 54 to 87 years. *Obesity (Silver Spring, Md.), 25*(3), 539–544. https://doi.org/10.1002/oby.21733

Jacobs, D. R., Pereira, M. A., Meyer, K. A., & Kushi, L. H. (2000). Fiber from whole grains, but not refined grains, is inversely associated with al-cause mortality in older women: the Iowa Women's Health Study. *Journal of the American College of Nutrition, 19*(sup3), 326S330S. https://doi.org/10.1080/07315724.2000.10718968

Janik, R., Thomason, L. A. M., Stanisz, A. M., Forsythe, P., Bienenstock, J., & Stanisz, G. J. (2016). Magnetic resonance spectroscopy reveals oral Lactobacillus promotion of increases in brain GABA, N-acetyl aspartate and glutamate. *NeuroImage, 125*, 988–995. https://doi.org/10.1016/j.neuroimage.2015.11.018

Javadivala, Z., Allahverdipour, H., Asghari Jafarabadi, M., & Emami, A. (2020). An Interventional strategy of physical activity promotion for reduction of menopause symptoms. *Health Promotion Perspectives, 10*(4), 383–392. https://doi.org/10.34172/hpp.2020.57

John Hopkins Medicine. (n.d.). *How sex changes after menopause.* John Hopkins Medicine. https://www.hopkinsmedicine.org/health/wellness-and-prevention/how-sex-changes-after-menopause

Johnson, K. (2020, February 26). *Menopause, an opportunity for new beginnings.* Live Well in WNC. https://livingwellwnc.com/menopause-an-opportunity/

Johnston, B. C., Kanters, S., Bandayrel, K., Wu, P., Naji, F., Siemieniuk, R. A., Ball, G. D. C., Busse, J. W., Thorlund, K., Guyatt, G., Jansen, J. P., & Mills, E. J. (2014). Comparison of weight loss among named diet programs in overweight and obese adults. *JAMA, 312*(9), 923. https://doi.org/10.1001/jama.2014.10397

Julian, J. (2023, March 29). *Makeup tips for mature skin from professional makeup artists.* Makeup.com. https://www.makeup.com/makeup-tutorials/expert-tips/mature-skin-makeup-tips

Kandiah, J., & Amend, V. (2010). An exploratory study on perceived relation-ship of alcohol, caffeine, and physical activity on hot flashes in menopausal women. *Health, 02*(09), 989–996. https://doi.org/10.4236/health.2010.29146

Kelly, J. R., Kennedy, P. J., Cryan, J. F., Dinan, T. G., Clarke, G., & Hyland, N. P. (2015). Breaking down the barriers: the gut microbiome, intestinal permeability and stress-related psychiatric disorders. *Frontiers in Cellular Neuroscience, 9*, 392. https://doi.org/10.3389/fncel.2015.00392

KINDRA. (n.d.). *The science of mental health during menopause.* KINDRA.

https://ourkindra.com/blogs/journal/the-science-of-mental-health-during-menopause

Kirby, S. (2023, October 30). *Menopause quotes about women's changing hormones.* Everyday Power. https://everydaypower.com/menopause-quotes/

König, D., Oesser, S., Scharla, S., Zdzieblik, D., & Gollhofer, A. (2018). Specific Collagen Peptides improve bone mineral density and bone markers in postmenopausal women—a randomized controlled study. *Nutrients, 10*(1), 97. https://doi.org/10.3390/nu10010097

Koothirezhi, R., & Ranganathan, S. (2021). *Postmenopausal syndrome.* PubMed; StatPearls Publishing. https://www.ncbi.nlm.nih.gov/books/NBK560840/

Kroenke, C. H., Caan, B. J., Stefanick, M. L., Anderson, G., Brzyski, R., Johnson, K. C., LeBlanc, E., Lee, C., La Croix, A. Z., Park, H. L., Sims, S. T., Vitolins, M., & Wallace, R. (2012). Effects of a dietary intervention and weight change on vasomotor symptoms in the Women's Health Initiative. *Menopause (New York, N.Y.), 19*(9), 980–988. https://doi.org/10.1097/gme.0b013e31824f606e

Kwon, S.-J., Ha, Y.-C., & Park, Y. (2017). High dietary sodium intake is associated with low bone mass in postmenopausal women: Korea National Health and Nutrition Examination Survey, 2008–2011. *Osteoporosis International, 28*(4), 1445–1452. https://doi.org/10.1007/s00198-017-3904-8

Lee, T. (2019, July 17). *How stress affects symptoms of menopause.* Healthspan. https://www.healthspan.co.uk/advice/mind/how-stress-affects-symptoms-of-menopause/

Lera Orsatti, F., Nahas, E. A., Maestá, N., Nahas Neto, J., Lera Orsatti, C., Vannucchi Portari, G., & Burini, R. C. (2014). Effects of resistance training frequency on body composition and metabolics and inflammatory markers in overweight postmenopausal women. *The Journal of Sports Medicine and Physical Fitness, 54*(3), 317–325. https://pubmed.ncbi.nlm.nih.gov/24739294/

Levine, B. (2019, May 2). *10 symptoms of menopause and perimenopause.* Everyday Health. https://www.everydayhealth.com/menopause/perimenopause-symptoms/

Lindberg, S. (2020, October 23). *Benefits and options for therapy.* Healthline. https://www.healthline.com/health/benefits-of-therapy#individual

Mackay, K. (n.d.). *It's never too late to reinvent yourself: 10 women who did it.*

CoveyClub. https://www.coveyclub.com/blog_posts/reinvent-yourself-10-women-who-did-it/

Mahon, A. K., Flynn, M. G., Stewart, L. K., McFarlin, B. K., Iglay, H. B., Mattes, R. D., Lyle, R. M., Considine, R. V., & Campbell, W. W. (2007). Protein intake during energy restriction: effects on body composition and markers of metabolic and cardiovascular health in postmenopausal women. *Journal of the American College of Nutrition, 26*(2), 182–189. https://doi.org/10.1080/07315724.2007.10719600

Mallett, J. (n.d.). *How a mindset can impact your life and help you learn more.* Beeline. https://www.beeline.life/buzz/how-a-mindset-can-impact-your-life-and-help-you-learn-more-5a65b

Manocha, R., Semmar, B., & Black, D. (2007). A pilot study of a mental silence form of meditation for women in perimenopause. *Journal of Clinical Psychology in Medical Settings, 14*(3), 266–273. https://doi.org/10.1007/s10880-007-9076-5

Maraboli, S. (n.d.). *Steve Maraboli quotes.* Goodreads. https://www.goodreads.com/quotes/507559-i-find-the-best-way-to-love-someone-is-not

Marketing Communication News. (2018, September 13). *Older women and menopause negatively stereotyped by the media, according to UM research.* Marketing Communication News. https://marcommnews.com/older-women-and-menopause-negatively-stereotyped-by-the-media-according-to-um-research/

The Marion Gluck Clinic. (2022, May 3). *Hormones and mental health - what's the connection?* The Marion Gluck Clinic. https://www.mariongluckclinic.com/blog/hormones-and-mental-health-whats-the-connection.html

Marmotta, G. (2022, November 8). *How to look & feel good during menopause!* LinkedIn. https://www.linkedin.com/pulse/how-look-feel-good-during-menopause-gessica-marmotta/?trk=pulse-article_more-articles_related-content-card

Mayo Clinic. (2023, May 25). *Menopause - Diagnosis and treatment.* Mayo Clinic. https://www.mayoclinic.org/diseases-conditions/menopause/diagnosis-treatment/drc-20353401

Mayo Clinic Staff . (2020, August 18). *Exercise and stress: Get moving to manage stress.* Mayo Clinic. https://www.mayoclinic.org/healthy-lifestyle/stress-management/in-depth/exercise-and-stress/art-20044469#:

Mayo Clinic Staff. (2023a, April 29). *Strength training: get stronger, leaner, healthier*. Mayo Clinic. https://www.mayoclinic.org/healthy-lifestyle/fitness/in-depth/strength-training/art-20046670#:

Mayo Clinic Staff. (2023b, July 8). *The reality of menopause weight gain*. Mayo Clinic. https://www.mayoclinic.org/healthy-lifestyle/womens-health/in-depth/menopause-weight-gain/art-20046058#:

McCullough, M. (2019, July 17). *Why does TV keep misrepresenting menopause?* Book and Film Globe. https://bookandfilmglobe.com/television/misrepresenting-menopause

McLaughlin, J. (2023, April 14). *Debunking the biggest myths about hormone replacement therapy*. Carrot. https://www.get-carrot.com/blog/debunking-the-biggest-myths-about-hormone-replacement-therapy

Mellberg, C., Sandberg, S., Ryberg, M., Eriksson, M., Brage, S., Larsson, C., Olsson, T., & Lindahl, B. (2014). Long-term effects of a Palaeolithic-type diet in obese postmenopausal women: a 2-year randomized trial. *European Journal of Clinical Nutrition, 68*(3), 350–357. https://doi.org/10.1038/ejcn.2013.290

Mental Health America. (n.d.). *Therapy*. Mental Health America. https://www.mhanational.org/therapy

Meyer, J. (n.d.). *Joyce Meyer quotes*. Quotespedia. https://www.quotespedia.org/authors/j/joyce-meyer/a-positive-attitude-gives-you-power-over-your-circumstances-instead-of-your-circumstances-having-power-over-you-joyce-meyer

Midlife Makeover. (2023, May 11). *Discover 10 unusual menopause symptoms you never knew existed*. Midlife Makeover. https://www.midlifemakeover.co.uk/blog/10-unusual-menopause-symptoms-you-never-knew-existed

Mirer, A. G., Young, T., Palta, M., Benca, R. M., Rasmuson, A., & Peppard, P. E. (2017). Sleep-disordered breathing and the menopausal transition among participants in the Sleep in Midlife Women Study. *Menopause, 24*(2), 157–162. https://doi.org/10.1097/gme.0000000000000744

Montare Behavioral Health. (2021, August 11). *The relationship between hormones and mental health*. Montare Behavioral Health. https://montarebehavioralhealth.com/the-relationship-between-hormones-and-mental-health/

Moore, J. (2020, November 25). *The history (and stigma) of menopause*. MenoMe. https://www.meno-me.com/the-history-and-stigma-of-menopause/

Mumusoglu, S., & Yildiz, B. O. (2019). Metabolic syndrome during menopause. *Current Vascular Pharmacology, 17*(6), 595–603. https://doi.org/10.2174/1570161116666180904094149

Munsi, P. (n.d.). *Menopause is not a disease. Experts call for new narrative for this natural stage of a woman's life.* CNN health. https://edition.cnn.com/2022/06/17/health/menopause-medicalization-women-ageing-bmj-as-equals-intl-cmd/index.html

Murtagh, M. J., & Hepworth, J. (2003). Menopause as a long-term risk to health: implications of general practitioner accounts of prevention for women's choice and decision-making. *Sociology of Health & Illness, 25*(2), 185–207. https://doi.org/10.1111/1467-9566.00331

Nash, J. (2016, April 14). *How to accept the impermanence of life: A Buddhist take.* PositivePsychology.com. https://positivepsychology.com/impermanence/

NBC News. (2005, December 16). Study: Key hormone therapy trial was flawed. *NBC News.* https://www.nbcnews.com/id/wbna10491951

Nhat Hanh. (n.d.). *Impermanence.* Facebook. https://m.facebook.com/ThichNhatHanhMindfulness/photos/impermanencenothing-remains-the-same-for-two-consecutive-moments-heraclitus-said/552076165141377/

NHS. (2023, February 8). *Benefits and risks of hormone replacement therapy (HRT).* NHS. https://www.nhs.uk/medicines/hormone-replacement-therapy-hrt/benefits-and-risks-of-hormone-replacement-therapy-hrt/

The North American Menopause Society. (n.d.-a). *Decreased desire.* The North American Menopause Society. https://www.menopause.org/for-women/sexual-health-menopause-online/sexual-problems-at-midlife/decreased-desire

The North American Menopause Society. (n.d.-b). *Hormone therapy: Benefits & risks.* The North American Menopause Society. https://www.menopause.org/for-women/menopauseflashes/menopause-symptoms-and-treatments/hormone-therapy-benefits-risks

The North American Menopause Society. (n.d.-c). *Make your menopause a positive experience.* The North American Menopause Society. https://www.menopause.org/for-women/menopauseflashes/menopause-symptoms-and-treatments/make-your-menopause-a-positive-experience

The North American Menopause Society. (2023a). *Depression, mood swings, anxiety.* North American Menopause Society. https://www.menopause.org/for-women/sexual-health-menopause-online/causes-of-sexual-problems/depression-mood-swings-anxiety

The North American Menopause Society. (2023b). *Pain with penetration.* North

American Menopause Society. https://www.menopause.org/for-women/sexual-health-menopause-online/sexual-problems-at-midlife/pain-with-penetration

Northeast Digestive. (2023, June 22). *The link between gut health & mental health.* Northeast Digestive. https://www.northeastdigestive.com/blog/the-link-between-gut-health-mental-health/

Northwestern Medicine. (2022, December). *Health benefits of having a routine.* Northwestern Medicine. https://www.nm.org/healthbeat/healthy-tips/health-benefits-of-having-a-routine#:

O'Mahony, S. M., Clarke, G., Borre, Y. E., Dinan, T. G., & Cryan, J. F. (2015). Serotonin, tryptophan metabolism and the brain-gut-microbiome axis. *Behavioural Brain Research, 277,* 32–48. https://doi.org/10.1016/j.bbr.2014.07.027

Oakley, C. (n.d.). *Guys' guide to menopause.* WebMD. https://www.webmd.com/menopause/features/guys-guide-menopause

Office on Women's Health. (2019, March 18). *Menopause basics.* Office on Women's Health. https://www.womenshealth.gov/menopause/menopause-basics

Olas, B. (2018). Berry phenolic antioxidants – implications for human health? *Frontiers in Pharmacology, 9.* https://doi.org/10.3389/fphar.2018.00078

Olson, E. J. (2023, February 21). *How many hours of sleep are enough for good health?* Mayo Clinic. https://www.mayoclinic.org/healthy-lifestyle/adult-health/expert-answers/how-many-hours-of-sleep-are-enough/faq-20057898

Oswal, Y. (2022, November 16). Impact of lifestyle on health. *The Times of India.* https://timesofindia.indiatimes.com/readersblog/wordsoul/impact-of-lifestyle-on-health-46692/

Pacheco, D. (2022, December 15). *How can menopause affect sleep?* Sleep Foundation. https://www.sleepfoundation.org/women-sleep/menopause-and-sleep

Parazzini, F. (2015). Resveratrol, tryptophanum, glycine and vitamin E: a nutraceutical approach to sleep disturbance and irritability in peri- and post-menopause. *Minerva Ginecologica, 67*(1). https://pubmed.ncbi.nlm.nih.gov/25660429/

Patade, A., Devareddy, L., Lucas, E. A., Korlagunta, K., Daggy, B. P., & Arjmandi, B. H. (2008). Flaxseed reduces total and LDL cholesterol concentrations in Native American postmenopausal women. *Journal of*

*Women's Health, 17*(3), 355–366. https://doi.org/10.1089/jwh.2007.0359

Pattemore, C. (2021, June 3). *10 ways to build and preserve better boundaries.* Psych Central. https://psychcentral.com/lib/10-way-to-build-and-preserve-better-boundaries#what-are-boundaries

Pellissier, S., Dantzer, C., Mondillon, L., Trocme, C., Gauchez, A.-S., Ducros, V., Mathieu, N., Toussaint, B., Fournier, A., Canini, F., & Bonaz, B. (2014). Relationship between vagal tone, cortisol, TNF-alpha, epinephrine and negative effects in Crohn's disease and irritable bowel syndrome. *PloS One, 9*(9), e105328. https://doi.org/10.1371/journal.pone.0105328

Powers, M. B., Asmundson, G. J. G., & Smits, J. A. J. (2015). Exercise for mood and anxiety disorders: The State-of-the Science. *Cognitive Behaviour Therapy, 44*(4), 237–239. https://doi.org/10.1080/16506073.2015.1047286

Purdue-Smithe, A. C., Whitcomb, B. W., Szegda, K. L., Boutot, M. E., Manson, J. E., Hankinson, S. E., Rosner, B. A., Troy, L. M., Michels, K. B., & Bertone-Johnson, E. R. (2017). Vitamin D and calcium intake and risk of early menopause. *The American Journal of Clinical Nutrition*, ajcn145607. https://doi.org/10.3945/ajcn.116.145607

Rains, T. M., Leidy, H. J., Sanoshy, K. D., Lawless, A. L., & Maki, K. C. (2015). A randomized, controlled, crossover trial to assess the acute appetitive and metabolic effects of sausage and egg-based convenience breakfast meals in overweight premenopausal women. *Nutrition Journal, 14*(1). https://doi.org/10.1186/s12937-015-0002-7

Raypole, C. (2020, November 13). *How to identify and manage your emotional triggers.* Healthline. https://www.healthline.com/health/mental-health/emotional-triggers

Rizzoli, R., Stevenson, J. C., Bauer, J. M., van Loon, L. J. C., Walrand, S., Kanis, J. A., Cooper, C., Brandi, M.-L., Diez-Perez, A., Reginster, J.-Y., & ESCEO Task Force. (2014). The role of dietary protein and vitamin D in maintaining musculoskeletal health in postmenopausal women: a consensus statement from the European Society for Clinical and Economic Aspects of Osteoporosis and Osteoarthritis (ESCEO). *Maturitas, 79*(1), 122–132. https://doi.org/10.1016/j.maturitas.2014.07.005

Robertson, R. (2023, July 31). *The gut-brain connection: how it works and the role of nutrition.* Healthline. https://www.healthline.com/nutrition/gut-brain-connection

Rodriguez, D. (2023, February 7). *Why exercise boosts mood and energy.* Everyday Health. https://www.everydayhealth.com/fitness/workouts/

boost-your-energy-level-with-exercise.aspx

Rohn, J. (n.d.). *Jim Rohn quotes.* BrainyQuote. https://www.brainyquote.com/quotes/jim_rohn_147499

Romagnolo, D. F., & Selmin, O. I. (2017). Mediterranean Diet and prevention of chronic diseases. *Nutrition Today, 52*(5), 208–222. https://doi.org/10.1097/nt.0000000000000228

Rowson, T. S., Jaworska, S., & Gibas, I. (2023). Hot topic: Examining discursive representations of menopause and work in the British media. *Gender, Work & Organization.* https://doi.org/10.1111/gwao.13021

Sabine Urgent Care. (2022, April 27). *How your lifestyle affects your general wellbeing.* abine Urgent Care. https://www.sabineurgentcare.com/blog/566851-how-your-lifestyle-affects-your-general-wellbeing/

Sackett-Fox, K., Gere, J., & Updegraff, J. (2021). Better together: The impact of exercising with a romantic partner. *Journal of Social and Personal Relationships, 38*(11), 026540752110120. https://doi.org/10.1177/02654075211012086

Santosa, S., & Jensen, M. D. (2012). Adipocyte fatty acid storage factors enhance subcutaneous fat storage in postmenopausal women. *Diabetes, 62*(3), 775–782. https://doi.org/10.2337/db12-0912

Sayón-Orea, C., Santiago, S., Cuervo, M., Martínez-González, M. A., Garcia, A., & Martínez, J. A. (2015). Adherence to Mediterranean dietary pattern and menopausal symptoms in relation to overweight/obesity in Spanish perimenopausal and postmenopausal women. *Menopause, 22*(7), 750–757. https://doi.org/10.1097/gme.0000000000000378

Scholey, A., & Owen, L. (2013). Effects of chocolate on cognitive function and mood: a systematic review. *Nutrition Reviews, 71*(10), 665–681. https://doi.org/10.1111/nure.12065

Schwartz, P. (2010, September). *A guy's guide to menopause - 6 tips on how to support the woman in your life.* AARP. https://www.aarp.org/relationships/love-sex/info-09-2010/naked_truth_men_guide_to_menopause.html

Scott, J. (2012, August 27). *A man's guide to menopause.* Everyday Health. EverydayHealth.com. https://www.everydayhealth.com/menopause/a-mans-guide-to-menopause.aspx

Secrets Boutiques. (n.d.). *What Is sensuality.* Secrets Boutiques. https://secretsboutiques.com/articles/what-is-sensuality/

Shaw, G. (n.d.). *Sensual vs. Sexual: What's the Difference.* WebMD. https://www.webmd.com/sex/features/sensual-vs-sexual

Silver, T. (2019, July 2). *Why is it important to exercise during menopause?* Beckwith Health Club. https://www.beckwithhealthclub.co.uk/exercise-during-menopause/

Simplyhealth. (2023). *Brain fog and the menopause.* Simplyhealth. https://www.simplyhealth.co.uk/healthy-living/womens-health/brain-fog

Singh, A. (2022, October 21). *How stereotypes affect middle-aged women's careers.* The Swaddle. https://theswaddle.com/how-stereotypes-affect-middle-aged-womens-careers/

Sliwinski, J. R., Johnson, A. K., & Elkins, G. R. (2014). Memory decline in peri- and post-menopausal women: the potential of mind–body medicine to improve cognitive performance. *Integrative Medicine Insights, 9,* IMI.S15682. https://doi.org/10.4137/imi.s15682

Snyder, C. (2022, June 29). *Diet and mental Health: Can what you eat affect how you feel?*Healthline. https://www.healthline.com/nutrition/diet-and-mental-health-can-what-you-eat-affect-how-you-feel

South African Menopause Society. (2019, November 13). *Midlife: A time of change and reflection.* South African Menopause Society. https://www.menopause.co.za/2019/11/13/a-time-of-change-and-reflection/

Spritzler, F. (2023, March 14). *How to lose weight around menopause (and keep it off).* Healthline. https://www.healthline.com/nutrition/lose-weight-in-menopause

Stefanopoulou, E., Shah, D., Shah, R., Gupta, P., Sturdee, D. W., & Hunter, M. S. (2013). An International Menopause Society study of Climate, Altitude, Temperature (IMS-CAT) and vasomotor symptoms in urban Indian regions. *Climacteric, 17*(4), 417–424. https://doi.org/10.3109/13697137.2013.852169

Steger, M. F. (2020, March 11). *Here's how to find meaning in your midlife crisis.* Greater Good Magazine. https://greatergood.berkeley.edu/article/item/heres_how_to_find_meaning_in_your_midlife_crisis

Stillman, J. (2021, January 7). *New research: Women leaders performed better during the Covid crisis. Empathy wins in a crisis.* Inc.Africa. https://incafrica.com/library/jessica-stillman-women-leaders-covid-jacinda-ardern

Suri, V., & Suri, V. (2014). Menopause and oral health. *Journal of Mid-Life Health, 5*(3), 115. https://doi.org/10.4103/0976-7800.141187

*10 surprising menopause symptoms.* (2023, April 26). Balance. https://www.balance-menopause.com/menopause-library/10-surprising-menopause-symptoms/

Terauchi, M., Horiguchi, N., Kajiyama, A., Akiyoshi, M., Owa, Y., Kato, K., & Kubota, T. (2014). Effects of grape seed proanthocyanidin extract on menopausal symptoms, body composition, and cardiovascular parameters in middle-aged women. *Menopause, 21*(9), 990–996. https://doi.org/10. 1097/gme.0000000000000200

Thompson, H. J., Sedlacek, S. M., Playdon, M. C., Wolfe, P., McGinley, J. N., Paul, D., & Lakoski, S. G. (2015). Weight loss interventions for breast cancer survivors: impact of dietary pattern. *PLOS ONE, 10*(5), e0127366. https://doi.org/10.1371/journal.pone.0127366

Torres, S. J., & Nowson, C. A. (2012). A moderate-sodium DASH-type diet improves mood in postmenopausal women. *Nutrition, 28*(9), 896–900. https://doi.org/10.1016/j.nut.2011.11.029

Turner-McGrievy, G. M., Barnard, N. D., & Scialli, A. R. (2007). A two-year randomized weight loss trial comparing a vegan diet to a more moderate low-fat diet*. *Obesity, 15*(9), 2276–2281. https://doi.org/10.1038/oby.2007.270

Upham, B. (2023, June 14). *Healthy foods for menopause*. Everyday Health. https://www.everydayhealth.com/menopause/healthy-foods-to-eat-during-menopause/

Valand, S. (2019, August 22). *How journaling can improve menopause symptoms*. Samantha Valand. https://samanthavaland.com/how-journaling-can-improve-menopause-symptoms/

Vázquez Cisneros, L. C., López-Uriarte, P., López-Espinoza, A., Navarro Meza, M., Espinoza-Gallardo, A. C., & Guzmán Aburto, M. B. (2017). Effects of green tea and its epigallocatechin (EGCG) content on body weight and fat mass in humans: a systematic review. *Nutricion Hospitalaria, 34*(3), 731–737. https://doi.org/10.20960/nh.753

Vitality. (2021, May 10). *How you can provide support to someone during menopause*. Vitality Magazine. https://magazine.vitality.co.uk/how-you-can-provide-support-to-someone-during-menopause/

Waltz, N. (2021, November 15). *The history of menopause*. Tabu. https://www.heytabu.com/blogs/mentionables/the-history-of-menopause

Ward Nutrition. (2020). *Midlife weight gain....sound familiar?* Ward Nutrition. https://www.wardnutrition.health/blog/midlife-weight-gainsound-familiar

Warren, J. M., Smith, N., & Ashwell, M. (2017). A structured literature review on the role of mindfulness, mindful eating and intuitive eating in changing eating behaviours: effectiveness and associated potential mechanisms. *Nutrition Research Reviews*, *30*(2), 272–283. https://doi.org/10.1017/s0954422417000154

Warrick, P. (1994, August 9). Feminists face off in war over menopause. *Los Angeles Times*. https://www.latimes.com/archives/la-xpm-1994-08-09-ls-25315-story.html

WebMD. (n.d.-a). *11 supplements for menopause symptoms*. WebMD. https://www.webmd.com/menopause/ss/slideshow-menopause

WebMD. (n.d.-b). *Depression overview slideshow*. WebMD. https://www.webmd.com/depression/ss/slideshow-depression-overview

WebMD Editorial Contributors. (n.d.). *Sex and Menopause*. WebMD. https://www.webmd.com/menopause/sex-menopause

Weiss, E. P., Jordan, R. C., Frese, E. M., Albert, S. G., & Villareal, D. T. (2017). Effects of weight loss on lean mass, strength, bone, and aerobic capacity. *Medicine & Science in Sports & Exercise*, *49*(1), 206–217. https://doi.org/10.1249/mss.0000000000001074

West, S. L. (2008). Prevalence of low sexual desire and hypoactive sexual desire disorder in a nationally representative sample of US women. *Archives of Internal Medicine*, *168*(13), 1441. https://doi.org/10.1001/archinte.168.13.1441

Wetmore, K. (2023, February 8). *Hormone replacement therapy: is Ii right for you?* Cedars-Sinai. https://www.cedars-sinai.org/blog/hormone-replacement-therapy-risks-benefits.html

Wild, S. (2023, February 1). *What's the best exercise for the menopause?* Bupa. https://www.bupa.co.uk/newsroom/ourviews/menopause-exercise

Withering Tendrils. (2021, May 26). *Impermanence*. Withering Tendrils. https://witheringtendrils.wordpress.com/2021/05/26/impermanence

Women's Health Network. (2023, February 27). *Menopause in different cultures*. Women's Health Network. https://www.womenshealthnetwork.com/menopause-and-perimenopause/menopause-in-different-cultures/

Women's Health Research Institute. (n.d.). *Menopause + hormone therapy*. Women's Health Research Institute. https://menopause.obgyn.msu.edu/

Wong, C. (2023, February 14). Evening primrose oil and menopause. Verywell Health. https://www.verywellhealth.com/evening-primrose-and-menopause-90067

Wright, L. (2023, March 16). *Sleep tips when you're in menopause*. Nuffield

Health. https://www.nuffieldhealth.com/article/sleep-tips-when-youre-in-menopause

Wu, R., Liu, L.-L., Zhu, H., Su, W.-J., Cao, Z.-Y., Zhong, S.-Y., Liu, X.-H., & Jiang, C.-L. (2019). Brief mindfulness meditation improves emotion processing. *Front. Neurosci, 13*. https://doi.org/10.3389/fnins.2019.01074

Yang, Y., Kim, Y., & Je, Y. (2018, December 1). *Fish consumption and risk of depression: epidemiological evidence from prospective studies.* Asia-Pacific Psychiatry: Official Journal of the Pacific Rim College of Psychiatrists. https://pubmed.ncbi.nlm.nih.gov/30238628/

Yano, J. M., Yu, K., Donaldson, G. P., Shastri, G. G., Ann, P., Ma, L., Nagler, C. R., Ismagilov, R. F., Mazmanian, S. K., & Hsiao, E. Y. (2015). Indigenous bacteria from the gut microbiota regulate host serotonin biosynthesis. *Cell, 161*(2), 264–276. https://doi.org/10.1016/j.cell.2015.02.047